Clinical Focus on
Fibroids

Clinical Focus on Fibroids

Series Editors

Neharika Malhotra
MD (Gold Medalist) DRM (Germany) DMIS FICMCH FMAS FICOG
ICOG Fellowship in Reproductive Medicine DGC
Consultant
Department of Obstetrics and Gynecology
Ujala Cygnus Rainbow Hospital
Agra, Uttar Pradesh, India

Jaideep Malhotra
MD FICOG FICS FIUMB FICMCH FMAS FRCPI FRCOG FICRM
Managing Director
ART Rainbow IVF Infertility
Agra, Uttar Pradesh, India

Narendra Malhotra
MD FIAJAGO FICMU FICOG FICMCH FRCOG FICS FMAS AFIAPM FICRM
Managing Director
Global Rainbow Health Care and MNMH (P) Ltd and
Ujala Cygnus Rainbow Hospital
Agra, Uttar Pradesh, India

Section Editors

Upma Saxena	**Shehla Jamal**
MD FICOG FICMCH	MBBS DNB
Professor, Consultant and Unit Head	Professor and Unit Head
Department of Obstetrics and Gynecology	Department of Obstetrics and Gynecology and
Vardhman Mahavir Medical College	Medical Education
and Safdarjung Hospital	Rajshree Medical Research Institute
New Delhi, India	Bareilly, Uttar Pradesh, India

Foreword
Sunita Tandulwadkar

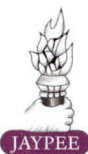

JAYPEE BROTHERS MEDICAL PUBLISHERS
The Health Sciences Publisher
New Delhi | London

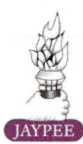

Jaypee Brothers Medical Publishers (P) Ltd

Headquarters
Jaypee Brothers Medical Publishers (P) Ltd
EMCA House, 23/23-B
Ansari Road, Daryaganj
New Delhi 110 002, India
Landline: +91-11-23272143, +91-11-23272703
+91-11-23282021, +91-11-23245672
Email: jaypee@jaypeebrothers.com

Corporate Office
Jaypee Brothers Medical Publishers (P) Ltd
4838/24, Ansari Road, Daryaganj
New Delhi 110 002, India
Phone: +91-11-43574357
Fax: +91-11-43574314
Email: jaypee@jaypeebrothers.com

Overseas Office
JP Medical Ltd.
83, Victoria Street, London
SW1H 0HW (UK)
Phone: +44 20 3170 8910
Fax: +44 (0)20 3008 6180
Email: info@jpmedpub.com

Website: www.jaypeebrothers.com
Website: www.jaypeedigital.com

© 2025, Jaypee Brothers Medical Publishers

The views and opinions expressed in this book are solely those of the original contributor(s)/author(s) and do not necessarily represent those of editor(s) or publisher of the book.

All rights reserved. No part of this publication may be reproduced, stored or transmitted in any form or by any means, electronic, mechanical, photocopying, recording or otherwise, without the prior permission in writing of the publishers.

All brand names and product names used in this book are trade names, service marks, trademarks or registered trademarks of their respective owners. The publisher is not associated with any product or vendor mentioned in this book.

Medical knowledge and practice change constantly. This book is designed to provide accurate, authoritative information about the subject matter in question. However, readers are advised to check the most current information available on procedures included and check information from the manufacturer of each product to be administered, to verify the recommended dose, formula, method and duration of administration, adverse effects and contraindications. It is the responsibility of the practitioner to take all appropriate safety precautions. Neither the publisher nor the author(s)/editor(s) assume any liability for any injury and/or damage to persons or property arising from or related to use of material in this book.

This book is sold on the understanding that the publisher is not engaged in providing professional medical services. If such advice or services are required, the services of a competent medical professional should be sought.

Every effort has been made where necessary to contact holders of copyright to obtain permission to reproduce copyright material. If any have been inadvertently overlooked, the publisher will be pleased to make the necessary arrangements at the first opportunity.

Inquiries for bulk sales may be solicited at: jaypee@jaypeebrothers.com

Clinical Focus on Fibroids

First Edition: **2025**

ISBN: 978-93-5696-631-4

Printed in India

Dedicated to

All the women who face the challenges of uterine fibroids with strength and resilience. We also honor the healthcare professionals whose unwavering commitment and expertise make a profound difference in women's health every day. Your dedication inspires us to continue striving for excellence in clinical care and research.

Contributors

Amrita Saha
MBBS MS FMAS MBA
Associate Professor and
Unit Head
Department of Obstetrics and
Gynecology
Government Medical College
Kannauj, Uttar Pradesh, India

Anshu Jindal
MD DNB MNAMS FICMCH
Reproductive Endocrinologist
Department of Infertility and
High-risk Obstetrics
Jindal Hospital and
Fertility Centre
Meerut, Uttar Pradesh, India

Apurba Kumar Dutta
MBBS MS (Gold Medalist) FIAOG
Assistant Professor
Department of Obstetrics and
Gynecology
IQ City Medical College and
Hospital
Durgapur, West Bengal, India

Aradhana Singh
MBBS MS FICOG FICMCH FGL PGDS
Additional Director
Department of Obstetrics and
Gynecology
Fortis Hospital
Noida, Uttar Pradesh, India

Aruna Nigam
MBBS MS FICOG FICMCH FMAS
MNAMS FIMSA
Professor and Head
Department of Obstetrics and
Gynecology
Hamdard Institute of Medical
Sciences and Research
New Delhi, India

Asma Khanday
MBBS MS
Assistant Professor
Department of Obstetrics and
Gynecology
Hamdard Institute of Medical
Sciences and Research
New Delhi, India

Deepali Raina
MBBS MD FAGOI FMAS
Associate Consultant
Department of Gynecologic
Oncology
Kokilaben Dhirubhai Ambani
Hospital
Mumbai, Maharashtra, India

Indranil Dutta
MBBS MS FIAOG FICOG FIAMS
PGDHHM PGDMLS
Professor and Unit Head
Department of Obstetrics and
Gynecology
IQ City Medical College
Durgapur, West Bengal, India

Jaideep Malhotra
MD FICOG FICS FIUMB FICMCH FMAS
FRCPI FRCOG FICRM
Managing Director
ART Rainbow IVF Infertility
Agra, Uttar Pradesh, India

Kavita Agarwal
DGO DNB MICOG FICOG FICMCH
Associate Professor
Department of Obstetrics and
Gynecology
Vardhman Mahavir Medical
College and
Safdarjung Hospital
New Delhi, India

Manpreet Sharma MBBS MS
Consultant
Department of Obstetrics and
Gynecology
Ujala Cygnus Rainbow Hospital
Agra, Uttar Pradesh, India

Mitra Saxena
MD DNB FICMCH FICOG Dip
Endoscopy (Kiel)
Medical Director and Head
Department of Obstetrics and
Gynecology
Shri Ashwini Saxena Hospital
Rewari, Haryana, India

Mohammad Noor A Alam
MBBS FCPS FRCS FACS
Professor
Department of Surgery
Ibrahim Medical College and
BIRDEM
Dhaka, Bangladesh

Monika Rana MBBS MS DNB
Senior Resident
Department of Obstetrics and
Gynecology
Vardhman Mahavir Medical
College and Safdarjung Hospital
New Delhi, India

Monisha Singh MBBS MD
Consultant
Department of Obstetrics and
Gynecology
Sarojini and Parul Hospital
Varanasi, Uttar Pradesh, India

Mousumi Das Ghosh
MD FICOG
Consultant
Department of Obstetrics and
Gynecology
Tata Main Hospital and Manipal
Tata Medical College
Jamshedpur, Jharkhand, India

Contributors

Mridula Sharma
MBBS DGO DNB FICMCH
Director and Consultant
Department of Obstetrics and Gynecology
Dharam Dutt City Hospital and Rajshree Medical Research Institute
Bareilly, Uttar Pradesh, India

Narendra Malhotra
MD FIAJAGO FICMU FICOG FICMCH FRCOG FICS FMAS AFIAPM FICRM
Managing Director
Global Rainbow Health Care and MNMH (P) Ltd and
Ujala Cygnus Rainbow Hospital
Agra, Uttar Pradesh, India

Neharika Malhotra
MD (Gold Medalist) DRM (Germany) DMIS FICMCH FMAS FICOG ICOG
Fellowship in Reproductive Medicine DGC
Consultant
Department of Obstetrics and Gynecology
Ujala Cygnus Rainbow Hospital
Agra, Uttar Pradesh, India

Parag Biniwale
MD FICOG
Chairman-Elect, ICOG
Consultant
Department of Obstetrics and Gynecology
Biniwale Clinic
Pune, Maharashtra, India

Parul Sinha
MBBS MS FICOG FICMCH FCCS (Obstetrics)
Associate Professor
Department of Obstetrics and Gynecology
All India Institute of Medical Sciences
Raebareli, Uttar Pradesh, India

Prerna Keshan
MBBS DGO FICOG FICMCH FIAOG
Consultant
Department of Obstetrics and Gynecology
Aditya Diagnostics and Hospital
Tinsukia, Assam, India

Rishu Goel
MBBS MD DNB
Senior Resident
Department of Obstetrics and Gynecology
All India Institute of Medical Sciences
New Delhi, India

Ruchika Garg
MS FICOG FICMCH FIMP FAMS
Editor-in-Chief
Journal of Midlife Health
Professor
Department of Obstetrics and Gynecology
SN Medical College
Agra, Uttar Pradesh, India

Sharmin Abbasi
MBBS MCPS FCPS FACS FART FMAS MSc (REI, UK)
Associate Professor
Department of Infertility and Obstetrics and Gynecology
Anwer Khan Modern Medical College Hospital
Dhaka, Bangladesh

Shehla Jamal
MBBS DNB
Professor and Unit Head
Department of Obstetrics and Gynecology and Medical Education
Rajshree Medical Research Institute
Bareilly, Uttar Pradesh, India

Shemi Bansal
MBBS Dip GO-ICMCH
Consultant
Department of Obstetrics and Gynecology
Ujala Cygnus Rainbow Hospital
Agra, Uttar Pradesh, India

Shivangini Varshney
MBBS MS
Senior Resident
Department of Obstetrics and Gynecology
Hamdard Institute of Medical Sciences and Research
New Delhi, India

Soniya Dhiman MBBS MD
Associate Professor
Department of Obstetrics and Gynecology
All India Institute of Medical Sciences
New Delhi, India

Subohi Khan MBBS MD
Assistant Professor
Department of Radiology
Hamdard Institute of Medical Sciences and Research
New Delhi, India

Upma Saxena
MD FICOG FICMCH
Professor, Consultant and Unit Head
Department of Obstetrics and Gynecology
Vardhman Mahavir Medical College and Safdarjung Hospital
New Delhi, India

Vijay Chandrakant Pawar
MD DNB (Obs and Gyne)
Associate Professor
Department of Obstetrics and Gynecology
Dr VM Government Medical College
Solapur, Maharashtra, India

Foreword

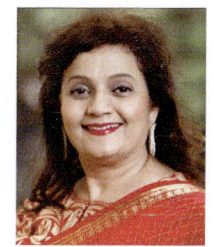

The *Clinical Focus on Fibroids* provides healthcare professionals with a comprehensive understanding of uterine fibroids, a prevalent gynecological condition affecting many women globally. This series explores the epidemiology, risk factors, classification, and advanced management options for fibroids, offering valuable insights for clinicians.

Fibroids, or leiomyomas, are benign tumors of the uterus and are most common in women of reproductive age. Their prevalence and impact on women's health make them a significant focus of clinical research and practice. The series begins with an in-depth examination of the epidemiology and risk factors associated with fibroids, laying the foundation for understanding their prevalence and implications.

The classification of fibroid uterus is systematically addressed, aiding in accurate diagnosis and categorization based on size, location, and symptomatology. Ultrasound assessment and differential diagnosis are crucial for identifying fibroids and distinguishing them from other uterine pathologies. The impact of fibroids on subfertility and abnormal uterine bleeding (AUB) patterns is explored, highlighting clinical challenges and management strategies.

Fibroid degeneration and calcification are examined alongside medical management options and presurgical hormonal treatments. The series also delves into surgical interventions, including laparoscopic, abdominal, and hysteroscopic myomectomy, with an emphasis on minimally invasive techniques.

Innovative treatments like the intrauterine system (IUS) and robotic-assisted management are presented as effective alternatives for fibroid management. The series also addresses the psychological and sexual dysfunctions associated with fibroids, ensuring a holistic approach to patient care.

Complex scenarios, including the management of recurrent fibroids, wandering and cervical fibroids, and challenges during cesarean sections, are examined. Additionally, the series covers rare conditions such as stromal tumors of uncertain malignant potential (STUMP) and atypical leiomyoma (ALM), providing a comprehensive guide for clinicians navigating these intricate issues.

I congratulate the Series Editors and Section Editors for publishing this essential handbook, a ready reckoner for every practicing gynecologist managing fibroids.

Sunita Tandulwadkar
President-Elect, FOGSI 2024

Preface

Clinical Focus on Fibroids is an illustrious manual about all the practical aspects for managing various pertinent challenges in day-to-day gynecological practice. Uterine fibroids, or leiomyomas, are the most prevalent benign tumors in women of reproductive age. Their effects range from subfertility and abnormal uterine bleeding (AUB) to significant psychological and sexual dysfunction, underscoring the urgent need for thorough understanding and effective management.

This clinical focus will not only help young clinicians for a ready-reckoner but also for seniors to update the topic with recent guidelines. This series begins with an exploration of the epidemiology and risk factors of fibroids, laying a foundation for clinicians to understand their varied presentations. The series then delve into the classification of fibroid uterus, facilitating accurate diagnosis and personalized treatment strategies based on size, location, and symptoms.

Key diagnostic tools, such as ultrasound assessment, are highlighted for their critical role in distinguishing fibroids from other uterine conditions. The series also examines the intricate link between fibroids and subfertility, emphasizing their impact on reproductive health.

Comprehensive management strategies for fibroids are explored, from medical management and presurgical hormonal treatments to various surgical interventions, including laparoscopic, abdominal, and hysteroscopic myomectomy. Special attention is given to complex scenarios, including recurrent fibroids, wandering and cervical fibroids, and challenges during cesarean sections. The series also addresses rare conditions like stromal tumors of uncertain malignant potential (STUMP) and atypical leiomyoma (ALM), providing clinicians with valuable insights into these complex issues. All the chapters have been thoroughly updated by incorporating guidelines and recent advances.

By presenting a holistic approach to fibroid management, this series aims to enhance clinical practice, improve patient outcomes, and support the ongoing education of healthcare professionals dedicated to women's health.

Upma Saxena
Shehla Jamal

Acknowledgments

It is with immense pleasure that we introduce the *Clinical Focus on Fibroids*. We begin by thanking the Almighty for His guidance and blessings in the successful creation and timely completion of this series.

We extend our heartfelt gratitude to Dr Sunita Tandulwadkar, who graciously agreed to write the "Foreword" for this book, providing us with her invaluable insights and perspectives.

Our profound thanks go to our esteemed mentors, Dr Narendra Malhotra, Dr Jaideep Malhotra, and Dr Niharika Malhotra. Their unwavering support, clinical wisdom, and academic excellence have been pivotal in assembling this comprehensive resource, especially beneficial for postgraduates and emerging clinical practitioners. Their enthusiasm and encouragement have continually inspired us.

We are deeply appreciative of the experts who responded promptly to our requests, contributing their knowledge and experience to each section, thereby blending the latest evidence with practical experience.

We also wish to acknowledge Shri Jitendar P Vij (Group Chairman), Mr Ankit Vij (Managing Director), and Ms Chetna Malhotra (Senior Director—Professional Publishing, Marketing, and Business Development) of M/s Jaypee Brothers Medical Publishers (P) Ltd, New Delhi, India, for their efforts in ensuring the timely publication of this book. Special thanks to Dr Sheeba Khan (Development Editor) for her meticulous attention and expertise in managing the final stages of editing.

This book is a result of collective efforts, where many experts have worked together to simplify complex concepts on fibroids into a comprehensive guide on fibroids, integrating evidence, guidelines, and practical insights in a clear and accessible manner.

We extend our special thanks to our colleagues and friends who supported our vision, motivated us to undertake this series and provided the confidence to see it through.

Lastly, we express our deepest gratitude to our families for their patience, understanding, and unwavering support during this endeavor.

Contents

1. **Understanding the Epidemiology and Risk Factors of Fibroids** 1
   Narendra Malhotra, Neharika Malhotra, Jaideep Malhotra,
   Manpreet Sharma, Shemi Bansal

2. **Classification of Fibroid Uterus** 19
   Sharmin Abbasi, Neharika Malhotra, Mohammad Noor A Alam

3. **Ultrasound Assessment and Differential Diagnosis of**
   Uterine Fibroids 28
   Aruna Nigam, Asma Khanday, Subohi Khan, Shivangini Varshney

4. **Fibroids and Subfertility** 34
   Anshu Jindal

5. **Fibroids and Abnormal Uterine Bleeding Patterns** 40
   Shehla Jamal

6. **Secondary Changes in Fibroid** 45
   Prerna Keshan

7. **Medical Management of Fibroids** 48
   Upma Saxena, Monika Rana

8. **Presurgical Hormonal Treatment** 62
   Vijay Chandrakant Pawar

9. **Laparoscopic Myomectomy** 65
   Parul Sinha

10. **Abdominal Myomectomy** 72
    Mitra Saxena

11. **Hysteroscopic Myomectomy** 80
    Kavita Agarwal

12. **Intrauterine System in Fibroids: An Effective Treatment Option** 84
    Parag Biniwale, Amrita Saha

13. **Sexual and Psychosexual Dysfunction** 88
    Monisha Singh, Neharika Malhotra

14. **Robotic-assisted Management of Fibroids** 92
    Indranil Dutta

15. **Management of Recurrent Fibroids** 96
    Mridula Sharma

16. **Wandering Fibroids** 102
    Soniya Dhiman, Rishu Goel

17. **Cervical Fibroids** 109
    Aradhana Singh

18. **Uterine-preserving Treatment Modalities** 114
    Apurba Kumar Dutta

19. **Challenges in Cesarean Section with Fibroids** 123
    Upma Saxena

20. **Uterine Smooth Muscle Tumors of Uncertain Malignant Potential** 130
    Deepali Raina

21. **Atypical Leiomyoma** 134
    Ruchika Garg, Mousumi Das Ghosh

Index *139*

CHAPTER 1

Understanding the Epidemiology and Risk Factors of Fibroids

Narendra Malhotra, Neharika Malhotra, Jaideep Malhotra, Manpreet Sharma, Shemi Bansal

■ INTRODUCTION

Fibroids, also known as uterine fibroids or leiomyomas, are noncancerous growths of the uterus that often appear during childbearing years. They can vary in size, ranging from as small as a seed to as large as a grapefruit.

These growths are composed of muscle and fibrous tissue and can develop either within the uterine wall, protrude into the uterine cavity, or extend outward from the uterus. While many women with fibroids experience no symptoms, others may have symptoms, such as heavy menstrual bleeding, prolonged menstrual periods, pelvic pressure or pain, frequent urination, difficulty emptying the bladder, or constipation.

The exact cause of fibroids is not well understood, but factors such as hormonal fluctuations, genetics, and ethnicity may play a role in their development.[1] Treatment options for fibroids depend on factors such as the size and location of the fibroids, the severity of symptoms, and whether the woman wishes to conceive in the future. Treatment options may include medication, minimally invasive procedures, or surgery such as a hysterectomy.

IMPORTANCE OF UNDERSTANDING EPIDEMIOLOGY AND RISK FACTORS

Understanding the epidemiology and risk factors associated with health conditions like fibroids is crucial for several reasons:[2]

- *Prevention and early detection:* Knowledge of risk factors allows healthcare providers to identify individuals who may be at a higher risk of developing fibroids. With this information, they can implement preventive measures or recommend screenings to detect fibroids at an early stage when treatment may be more effective.
- *Tailored interventions:* Understanding the epidemiology and risk factors helps in designing tailored interventions for different population groups. For example, if certain demographic groups or lifestyle factors are associated with a higher risk of fibroids, interventions can be targeted toward those groups to promote awareness, lifestyle modifications, or early screening.
- *Resource allocation:* By understanding the prevalence of fibroids and the

populations most affected, healthcare resources can be allocated more efficiently. This includes directing funding toward research, prevention efforts, and healthcare services in areas with higher prevalence rates or among populations with increased risk factors.

- *Health equity:* Epidemiological studies can uncover disparities in the prevalence and management of fibroids among different demographic groups. This knowledge is essential for addressing health inequities and ensuring that all individuals have access to appropriate prevention, diagnosis, and treatment options.
- *Advancing research:* Epidemiological data provides a foundation for further research into the causes, mechanisms, and optimal management of fibroids. By identifying trends and associations, researchers can delve deeper into understanding the underlying biology of fibroids and develop new therapeutic approaches.
- *Patient education and empowerment:* Knowledge of risk factors empowers individuals to take proactive steps to reduce their risk of developing fibroids. Through education and awareness campaigns, individuals can learn about lifestyle modifications, reproductive health choices, and symptom recognition, enabling them to make informed decisions about their health.

Prevalence

Global Prevalence Rates

Estimating the global prevalence rates of uterine fibroids can be challenging due to variations in reporting methods, healthcare access, and population demographics across different regions. However, fibroids are a common gynecological condition, particularly among women of reproductive age. Prevalence rates may also vary based on factors such as ethnicity, genetic predisposition, and lifestyle factors. A general overview is as follows:

- *Overall prevalence:* Uterine fibroids are estimated to affect between 20% and 80% of women by the age of 50 years. However, the exact prevalence varies widely across populations and studies.
- *Ethnic and racial disparities:* There are significant ethnic and racial disparities in the prevalence of fibroids. For example, studies have shown that Black women tend to have a higher prevalence of fibroids and may experience more severe symptoms compared to women of other racial or ethnic groups.[1]
- *Geographic variations:* Prevalence rates may also differ based on geographic regions. While fibroids are common in developed countries, they may be less frequently reported in some developing regions due to differences in healthcare access, diagnostic methods, and reporting practices.
- *Age and reproductive status:* Fibroids are more common in women of reproductive age, particularly between the ages of 30 and 50 years. The prevalence tends to decrease after menopause when estrogen levels decline.
- *Impact of risk factors:* Certain risk factors, such as nulliparity (never having given birth), early onset of menstruation, obesity, and a family history of fibroids, may increase the likelihood of developing fibroids. Regions or populations with higher prevalence rates of these risk factors may also have higher overall prevalence rates of fibroids.
- *Economic and healthcare factors:* Access to healthcare services and diagnostic tools

can influence the detection and reporting of fibroids. In regions with limited access to healthcare, under-reporting of fibroids may occur, leading to underestimated prevalence rates.

While precise global prevalence rates may be difficult to ascertain, it is clear that uterine fibroids represent a significant public health concern worldwide, impacting the quality of life and reproductive health of millions of women. Further research and efforts to improve awareness, access to healthcare, and treatment options are essential to address the burden of fibroids on a global scale.

Variation Among Different Populations

Variation in the prevalence of uterine fibroids among different populations can be influenced by a variety of factors, including genetics, ethnicity, lifestyle, reproductive history, and access to healthcare. How these factors contribute to variations is given in the following text:

- *Ethnicity and race:* There are notable differences in the prevalence of fibroids among ethnic and racial groups. Studies have consistently shown that Black women have a higher prevalence of fibroids compared to women of other racial or ethnic backgrounds. For example, in the United States, Black women are two to three times more likely to develop fibroids than White women. Hispanic and Asian women also have intermediate prevalence rates compared to Black and White women.[1]
- *Genetic predisposition:* Genetic factors play a significant role in the development of fibroids. Certain genetic variations and susceptibility genes have been identified that may increase the risk of fibroids. These genetic factors can vary among populations and contribute to differences in fibroid prevalence.
- *Reproductive factors:* Reproductive factors, such as parity (number of pregnancies), age at first childbirth, and use of hormonal contraceptives, can influence the risk of fibroids. Women who have never given birth (nulliparous) or had their first child at a later age may have a higher risk of fibroids. Differences in reproductive patterns among populations can contribute to variations in fibroid prevalence.[2]
- *Hormonal and lifestyle factors:* Hormonal factors, such as estrogen and progesterone levels, play a key role in the growth of fibroids. Lifestyle factors such as obesity, diet, and physical activity can also influence hormone levels and contribute to fibroid development. Variations in lifestyle behaviors among populations may impact fibroid prevalence.
- *Access to healthcare and diagnostic practices:* Disparities in access to healthcare, including preventive care and diagnostic imaging, can affect the detection and reporting of fibroids. In some populations or regions with limited healthcare resources, fibroids may be underdiagnosed or untreated, leading to lower reported prevalence rates.
- *Environmental factors:* Environmental exposures, such as endocrine-disrupting chemicals (EDCs) and pollutants, have been implicated in the development of fibroids. Variations in environmental exposures among populations may contribute to differences in fibroid prevalence.

Trends Over Time

Over time, several trends regarding uterine fibroids have been observed, influenced by changes in healthcare practices, demographics, lifestyle factors, and awareness. Some notable trends are as follows:

- *Increased awareness and diagnosis:* Awareness of uterine fibroids has grown over time, leading to increased diagnosis and reporting of the condition. Improved imaging techniques and greater awareness among healthcare providers and patients have contributed to earlier detection and diagnosis of fibroids.
- *Changing demographics:* Changes in demographics, including aging populations and shifts in racial and ethnic composition, can influence the prevalence of fibroids. For example, as populations age, the prevalence of fibroids among postmenopausal women may decline due to decreasing estrogen levels. However, the overall burden of fibroids may still increase due to population growth and changes in reproductive patterns.
- *Advancements in treatment options:* Over the years, there have been advancements in the treatment of fibroids, including minimally invasive procedures, such as laparoscopic or robotic surgery, uterine artery embolization, and MRI-guided focused ultrasound surgery. These advancements have provided more options for women seeking treatment, potentially impacting trends in fibroid management and outcomes.
- *Healthcare disparities:* Disparities in access to healthcare and treatment remain a concern, particularly among underserved populations and minority groups. Efforts to address healthcare disparities and improve access to care may impact trends in fibroid prevalence and outcomes over time.
- *Impact of lifestyle factors:* Changes in lifestyle factors, such as obesity rates, diet, and physical activity levels, can influence hormone levels and the development of fibroids. Increasing rates of obesity, for example, may contribute to a higher prevalence of fibroids in certain populations. Increased dairy intake and risk of fibroid have also been documented.[3]
- *Research and education initiatives:* Ongoing research efforts and educational campaigns aimed at increasing awareness of fibroids, promoting preventive measures, and advancing treatment options can influence trends over time. Increased knowledge and understanding of fibroids among both healthcare providers and the general population may lead to improvements in diagnosis, management, and outcomes.
- *Globalization and urbanization:* Globalization and urbanization have led to changes in lifestyle and environmental factors that may impact fibroid prevalence. Urban environments may be associated with higher stress levels, sedentary lifestyles, and exposure to environmental pollutants, which could potentially influence fibroid development.

Incidence

Incidence Patterns

The incidence patterns of uterine fibroids, or the rate at which new cases of fibroids occur within a population over time, can vary based on several factors. Some key patterns observed in the incidence of uterine fibroids are as follows:

- *Age-specific incidence:* The incidence of fibroids tends to increase with age, peaking during the reproductive years and declining after menopause. Fibroids are most commonly diagnosed in women

aged 30–50 years, although they can occur at any age. The age-specific incidence reflects the hormonal influences on fibroid development, as estrogen and progesterone levels fluctuate throughout a woman's reproductive life.[4]
- *Racial and ethnic disparities:* Studies have consistently shown disparities in the incidence of fibroids among different racial and ethnic groups. For example, Black women have been found to have a higher incidence of fibroids compared to White women. Hispanic and Asian women also have intermediate incidence rates. These disparities may be influenced by genetic factors, hormonal differences, and socioeconomic factors.
- *Reproductive history:* A complete reproductive history should be taken and documented as stated above reproductive factors impact incidence and outcome of fibroids. Additionally, hormonal contraceptive use, particularly combined oral contraceptives (COCs), has been associated with a reduced risk of fibroids.[5]
- *Geographic and environmental factors:* Incidence patterns of fibroids may vary geographically and be influenced by environmental factors, such as diet, lifestyle, and exposure to EDCs. Urban environments, for example, may be associated with higher rates of fibroids due to factors such as stress, obesity, and pollution.
- *Advancements in diagnostic techniques:* The incidence of fibroids may be influenced by improvements in diagnostic techniques, leading to increased detection of asymptomatic cases. The widespread use of imaging modalities, such as ultrasound, magnetic resonance imaging (MRI), and hysteroscopy, has facilitated the detection of fibroids, potentially impacting incidence rates over time.
- *Changing healthcare practices:* Changes in healthcare practices, including increased access to healthcare, routine screenings, and preventive care, may also influence the incidence of fibroids. Greater awareness among healthcare providers and patients, as well as advancements in treatment options, may lead to earlier diagnosis and management of fibroids, affecting incidence patterns.

Factors Influencing Incidence Rates

Several factors influence the incidence rates of uterine fibroids, contributing to the development of this common gynecological condition. Some key factors are as follows:
- *Hormonal factors:* Hormones, particularly estrogen and progesterone, play a central role in the development and growth of fibroids. Fibroids often grow during the reproductive years when hormone levels are high and tend to shrink after menopause when hormone levels decline. Factors that affect hormone levels, such as hormonal contraceptives, hormone replacement therapy (HRT), and hormonal fluctuations during the menstrual cycle, can influence the incidence of fibroids.
- *Genetic predisposition:* Genetic factors contribute to an individual's susceptibility to fibroids. Family history studies have shown that women with a family history of fibroids are at an increased risk of developing them. Specific genetic variations and susceptibility genes associated with fibroids have been identified, although the exact genetic mechanisms underlying fibroid development are still being elucidated.

- *Reproductive history:* Reproductive factors, such as nulliparity (never having given birth), late age at first childbirth, and infertility, are associated with an increased risk of fibroids. Conversely, factors that reduce lifetime estrogen exposure, such as early childbirth and prolonged breastfeeding, may decrease the risk of fibroids. The number of pregnancies and hormonal changes during pregnancy can also influence fibroid incidence.
- *Race and ethnicity:* There are significant racial and ethnic disparities in the incidence of fibroids, with Black women having the highest incidence rates compared to women of other racial and ethnic groups. Hispanic and Asian women also have intermediate incidence rates, while White women have the lowest rates. The reasons for these disparities are multifactorial and likely involve a combination of genetic, hormonal, and environmental factors.
- *Obesity:* This is associated with an increased risk of fibroids, possibly due to alterations in hormone metabolism and increased estrogen levels in obese individuals. A higher body mass index (BMI) is consistently associated with a greater risk of developing fibroids, and weight loss may reduce the risk or slow the growth of fibroids in some cases.
- *Lifestyle factors:* Certain lifestyle factors, such as diet, physical activity, and stress, may influence the incidence of fibroids. Diets high in red meat, processed foods, and sugar and low in fruits, vegetables, and fiber have been associated with a higher risk of fibroids. Regular physical activity and stress reduction techniques may help lower the risk of fibroids by modulating hormone levels and reducing inflammation.
- *Environmental exposures:* Exposure to environmental factors, such as EDCs [e.g., phthalates, bisphenol A (BPA)] and pollutants, may contribute to the development of fibroids. These chemicals can mimic or interfere with hormones in the body, potentially promoting the growth of fibroids.
- *Healthcare access and screening practices:* Disparities in healthcare access and screening practices can affect the detection and diagnosis of fibroids, potentially influencing reported incidence rates. Women with limited access to healthcare may have undiagnosed fibroids or delayed diagnosis, leading to underestimation of incidence rates in certain populations.

Demographic Patterns

Age Distribution

The incidence and prevalence of uterine fibroids vary across different age groups, reflecting the influence of hormonal changes, reproductive factors, and other demographic characteristics. How age distribution typically affects the occurrence of uterine fibroids is as follows:[6]

- *Reproductive age:* Uterine fibroids are most commonly diagnosed during the reproductive years, typically between the ages of 30 and 50 years. During this period, hormone levels, particularly estrogen and progesterone, are at their highest, which may contribute to the growth and development of fibroids. As a result, fibroids are more prevalent among women of reproductive age compared to other age groups.
- *Peak incidence:* The highest incidence of uterine fibroids is typically observed in women in their 40s, although fibroids can develop at any point during the

reproductive years. Studies have shown that the incidence of fibroids increases with age until around the age of 45–50 years and then stabilizes or declines after menopause. This age-related pattern reflects the influence of hormonal changes and reproductive factors on fibroid development.

- *Perimenopausal transition:* The perimenopausal transition, which occurs in the years leading up to menopause, is a period of hormonal fluctuation and changes in menstrual patterns. During this time, fibroids may continue to grow or cause symptoms in some women, while in others, fibroids may stabilize or shrink due to declining estrogen levels. The incidence of fibroids may vary among women in the perimenopausal age-group, with some experiencing worsening symptoms while others may have symptom relief.
- *Postmenopausal period:* After menopause, when estrogen levels decline, the incidence of fibroids generally decreases. Fibroids may shrink or become less symptomatic in postmenopausal women, although they may still be present. The prevalence of fibroids among postmenopausal women is lower compared to women of reproductive age, reflecting the hormonal changes associated with menopause.
- *Age-related symptoms:* While fibroids may develop at any age during the reproductive years, they are more likely to cause symptoms such as heavy menstrual bleeding, pelvic pain, and pressure-related symptoms (e.g., urinary frequency, constipation) in older women. This is because fibroids tend to grow larger over time and may become symptomatic as women age.

Gender Distribution

Uterine fibroids primarily affect individuals assigned female at birth (AFAB) as they develop in the uterus. Therefore, the gender distribution of uterine fibroids is overwhelmingly skewed toward individuals who have a uterus, typically women. While fibroids can occur rarely in individuals with certain intersex variations or transgender men who have retained their uterus, the vast majority of cases occur in cisgender women.

As fibroids develop within the uterine tissue, their presence and potential impact on health are limited to individuals with a uterus. Therefore, the gender distribution of uterine fibroids is inherently tied to biological sex and the presence of female reproductive anatomy. However, it is important to recognize that gender identity and expression are distinct from biological sex, and individuals of diverse gender identities may be affected by fibroids if they have a uterus.

In summary, uterine fibroids predominantly affect individuals AFAB, reflecting their development within the uterus. While gender distribution aligns with biological sex in this context, it is crucial to acknowledge the diversity of gender identities and experiences among those affected by fibroids.

Ethnic and Racial Disparities

Ethnic and racial disparities in uterine fibroids' prevalence and outcomes are well documented, with significant differences observed among various racial and ethnic groups. An overview of these disparities is as follows:

- *Higher prevalence in Black women:* Black women have the highest reported prevalence of uterine fibroids compared to other racial and ethnic groups. Studies

consistently show that Black women are two to three times more likely to develop fibroids than White women. Fibroids in Black women also tend to occur at younger ages, grow larger, and cause more severe symptoms.
- *Intermediate prevalence in Hispanic and Asian women:* Hispanic and Asian women have intermediate prevalence rates of uterine fibroids compared to Black and White women. While the prevalence of fibroids in these groups is lower than that of Black women, it is higher than that of White women. Studies have shown variations in fibroid prevalence among different Hispanic subgroups.
- *Lower prevalence in White women:* White women have the lowest reported prevalence of uterine fibroids compared to other racial and ethnic groups. However, fibroids still affect a significant proportion of White women, particularly as they age.
- *Impact on health disparities:* Fibroids contribute to health disparities, affecting various aspects of a woman's health and well-being. Black women with fibroids are more likely to experience symptoms, such as heavy menstrual bleeding, pelvic pain, and reproductive health issues compared to White women. Fibroids in Black women also tend to be diagnosed at more advanced stages and may require more invasive treatments.
- *Socioeconomic and healthcare access factors:* Socioeconomic factors, including income, education, and access to healthcare, contribute to racial and ethnic disparities in fibroid prevalence and outcomes. Black women are more likely to experience socioeconomic disadvantages and barriers to healthcare access, which can impact the timely diagnosis and management of fibroids.
- *Genetic and biological factors:* While genetic factors likely play a role in racial and ethnic disparities in fibroid prevalence, the exact mechanisms are not fully understood. Studies have identified genetic variations associated with fibroids that may contribute to differences in susceptibility among racial and ethnic groups. Additionally, biological differences in hormone metabolism and immune function may influence fibroid development and growth.

■ RISK FACTORS FOR FIBROIDS

Genetic Factors

Familial Predisposition

Familial predisposition to uterine fibroids suggests a genetic component in the development of this condition. How genetic factors contribute to familial predisposition is as follows:
- *Family history:* Women with a family history of uterine fibroids are at an increased risk of developing them themselves. Having a first-degree relative (such as a mother or sister) with fibroids significantly increases a woman's risk of also developing fibroids. This suggests that genetic factors passed down through families play a role in fibroid development.
- *Genetic studies:* Several genetic studies have identified variations in specific genes associated with an increased risk of uterine fibroids. While the exact genetic mechanisms underlying fibroid development are still being elucidated, researchers have identified candidate genes involved in processes such as cell proliferation, hormone receptor signaling, extracellular matrix regulation, and inflammation. Variations in these

genes may contribute to an individual's susceptibility to fibroids.
- *Polygenic inheritance:* Uterine fibroids are considered a complex, polygenic disorder, meaning that multiple genetic variations across different genes likely contribute to an individual's risk of developing fibroids. These genetic variations may interact with environmental factors and hormonal influences to influence fibroid development.
- *Ethnic and racial differences*: Genetic studies have also revealed ethnic and racial differences in the genetic risk factors associated with fibroids. Certain genetic variations may be more prevalent or have stronger effects in certain racial or ethnic groups, contributing to the observed disparities in fibroid prevalence among different populations.
- *Gene–environment interactions:* While genetic factors play a significant role in fibroid development, they do not fully explain the variations in fibroid prevalence observed among different individuals and populations. Gene–environment interactions, such as exposure to EDCs, diet, lifestyle factors, and reproductive history, also influence fibroid risk. These environmental factors may interact with genetic predispositions to modulate an individual's susceptibility to fibroids.

Candidate Genes Associated with Fibroids

Several candidate genes have been identified as potentially associated with uterine fibroids through genetic studies. These genes are involved in various biological processes, including cell proliferation, hormone receptor signaling, extracellular matrix regulation, and inflammation. While the exact role of each gene in fibroid development is still being elucidated, some examples of candidate genes associated with fibroids are as follows:

- *COL4A5 (collagen type IV alpha 5):* COL4A5 encodes a component of type IV collagen, a major structural protein in the extracellular matrix. Variations in COL4A5 have been associated with an increased risk of fibroids, possibly due to alterations in extracellular matrix regulation and tissue remodeling processes.
- *MED12 (mediator complex subunit 12):* MED12 is a component of the mediator complex, which regulates gene expression by facilitating interactions between transcription factors and RNA polymerase II. Mutations in MED12 have been found in a subset of fibroids, particularly those with a specific histological subtype called "uterine leiomyoma with MED12 mutation." MED12 mutations may contribute to abnormal cell proliferation and growth in fibroids.
- *HMGA2 (high mobility group AT-Hook 2):* HMGA2 is involved in chromatin remodeling and transcriptional regulation. Variations in HMGA2 have been associated with an increased risk of fibroids, possibly through effects on cell proliferation and differentiation.
- *FSHR (follicle-stimulating hormone receptor):* FSHR encodes the follicle-stimulating hormone receptor, which is involved in ovarian function and hormone signaling. Variations in FSHR have been implicated in fibroid development, potentially through effects on hormone receptor signaling and ovarian function.
- *ESR1 (estrogen receptor 1)* and *ESR2 (estrogen receptor 2):* Estrogen receptors play a critical role in mediating the effects of estrogen on target tissues, including the uterus. Variations in ESR1 and ESR2 have been associated with an increased risk of fibroids, suggesting that dysregulation

of estrogen signaling pathways may contribute to fibroid development.
- *CYP19A1 (cytochrome P450 family 19 subfamily A member 1):* CYP19A1 encodes aromatase, an enzyme involved in estrogen biosynthesis. Variations in *CYP19A1* have been linked to fibroid risk, potentially through effects on estrogen production and metabolism.
- *COL1A1 (collagen type I alpha 1)* and *COL3A1 (collagen type III alpha 1):* Collagen genes, including *COL1A1* and *COL3A1*, are involved in extracellular matrix remodeling and tissue structure. Variations in these genes have been associated with fibroid risk, possibly through effects on tissue integrity and remodeling processes.

These are just a few examples of candidate genes associated with uterine fibroids. Research into the genetic basis of fibroids is ongoing, and additional genes and genetic pathways may be implicated in fibroid development as our understanding of the condition continues to evolve.

Genetic Susceptibility Studies

Genetic susceptibility studies aim to identify genetic variations or mutations associated with an increased risk of developing uterine fibroids. These studies typically involve analyzing the DNA of individuals with and without fibroids to identify genetic differences that may contribute to fibroid risk. An overview of genetic susceptibility studies conducted in the field of uterine fibroids is as follows:

- *Genome-wide association studies (GWAS):* GWAS are large-scale studies that analyze hundreds of thousands to millions of genetic variations across the entire genome to identify common genetic variants associated with fibroid risk. GWAS have identified several genetic loci associated with fibroids, including variations in genes involved in cell proliferation, hormone signaling, and extracellular matrix regulation.
- *Candidate gene studies:* Candidate gene studies focus on specific genes or genetic pathways implicated in fibroid development based on biological knowledge or previous research findings. These studies typically involve comparing the frequency of genetic variations in candidate genes between individuals with and without fibroids to identify potential associations with fibroid risk.
- *Exome sequencing and whole-genome sequencing:* Exome sequencing and whole-genome sequencing are comprehensive sequencing techniques that analyze the protein-coding regions of the genome (exome) or the entire genome (whole genome) to identify rare genetic variants or mutations associated with fibroid risk. These studies may uncover rare genetic mutations in genes involved in fibroid pathogenesis.
- *Family-based studies:* Family-based studies examine the inheritance patterns of fibroids within families to identify genetic factors contributing to familial predisposition. These studies may involve analyzing genetic data from multiple affected and unaffected family members to identify genetic variations segregating with fibroid risk within families.
- *Functional studies:* These aim to elucidate the biological mechanisms underlying genetic associations with fibroids. These studies may involve laboratory experiments to assess the functional effects of genetic variations on cellular processes relevant to fibroid development, such as cell proliferation, hormone signaling, and extracellular matrix remodeling.

- *Meta-analysis and replication studies:* Meta-analysis and replication studies combine data from multiple genetic susceptibility studies to validate and replicate findings across different populations. These studies help confirm the association of specific genetic variants with fibroid risk and identify genetic loci with robust and consistent effects across diverse populations.

Hormonal Factors

Estrogen and progesterone play crucial roles in the development and growth of uterine fibroids. How these hormones influence fibroid growth as well as the relationship between hormonal therapies and fibroid risk is as follows:

- *Role of estrogen and progesterone:*
  - *Estrogen:* It stimulates the growth and proliferation of uterine cells, including those in fibroids. Estrogen receptors are present in fibroid cells, and estrogen binding to these receptors can promote cell division and fibroid growth.
  - *Progesterone:* Progesterone, another female sex hormone, also plays a role in fibroid growth. Progesterone receptors are expressed in fibroid tissues, and progesterone signaling can contribute to fibroid development by promoting cell proliferation and inhibiting cell death (apoptosis).
- *Hormonal fluctuations and fibroid growth:* Hormonal fluctuations during the menstrual cycle, pregnancy, and menopause can influence fibroid growth. Fibroids tend to grow in response to increased levels of estrogen and progesterone during the reproductive years.

  Fibroids may increase in size during pregnancy due to elevated hormone levels, but they may shrink after menopause when hormone levels decline. However, fibroids may continue to cause symptoms in some women even after menopause.
- *Hormonal therapies and fibroid risk:*
  - *Hormonal contraceptives:* COCs containing estrogen and progestin have been associated with a reduced risk of fibroids. These hormonal contraceptives suppress ovulation and reduce the production of endogenous estrogen and progesterone, which may help prevent fibroid growth.
  - Hormone replacement therapy (HRT) can have significant effects on uterine fibroids, which are non-cancerous growths in the uterus. Using a combination of estrogen and progestogen can sometimes help mitigate the growth-promoting effects of estrogen on fibroids.
  - *Selective estrogen receptor modulators (SERMs):* SERMs are a class of medications that modulate estrogen receptor activity. While some SERMs have been investigated for their potential use in treating fibroids, their efficacy and safety for this indication are still under evaluation.

In summary, estrogen and progesterone play pivotal roles in the development and growth of uterine fibroids. Hormonal fluctuations during the menstrual cycle, pregnancy, and menopause can influence fibroid growth. Hormonal therapies, such as hormonal contraceptives, HRT, and SERMs, may impact fibroid risk and growth by modulating hormone levels and receptor activity. However, the effects of these therapies on fibroids can vary among individuals, and careful consideration of the risks and benefits is essential when prescribing hormonal treatments for women with fibroids.

Reproductive Factors

Reproductive factors such as parity (number of pregnancies), age at menarche (onset of menstruation), age at menopause, and fertility treatments can influence the risk of developing uterine fibroids and their clinical course. How these factors relate to fibroids is as follows:

- *Parity and pregnancy:*
  - *Parity:* Studies have shown that parity, or the number of pregnancies a woman has had, is inversely associated with the risk of developing fibroids. Women who have had more pregnancies, especially full-term pregnancies, tend to have a lower risk of fibroids compared to nulliparous women. The protective effect of parity may be attributed to hormonal changes and alterations in uterine structure that occur during pregnancy.
  - *Pregnancy:* This can have varying effects on fibroids. In some cases, fibroids may increase in size during pregnancy due to hormonal changes and increased blood flow to the uterus. Fibroids may also cause complications during pregnancy, such as miscarriage, preterm birth, or breech presentation. However, in other cases, fibroids may remain stable or even decrease in size after pregnancy, particularly following childbirth and breastfeeding.
- *Age at menarche and menopause:*
  - *Age at menarche:* Early age at menarche (onset of menstruation) has been associated with an increased risk of fibroids. Early menarche is thought to reflect longer exposure to estrogen over a woman's reproductive lifespan, which may contribute to the development of fibroids.
  - *Age at menopause:* The risk of fibroids tends to decrease after menopause when estrogen levels decline. Women who reach menopause at an older age may have a longer duration of estrogen exposure and may be at a slightly higher risk of developing fibroids compared to women who reach menopause at a younger age. However, fibroids can still cause symptoms in postmenopausal women and may require management.
- *Impact of fertility treatments:*
  - *Assisted reproductive technologies (ART):* Fertility treatments such as in vitro fertilization (IVF) and ovulation induction may influence the risk of fibroids or exacerbate existing fibroids. While the evidence is mixed, some studies suggest that fertility treatments, particularly gonadotropin stimulation used in IVF, may increase the risk of fibroids or lead to their growth. However, other factors, such as underlying infertility and hormonal factors associated with fertility treatments, may also contribute to fibroid risk.

Reproductive factors play a significant role in the development and clinical course of uterine fibroids. Understanding how parity, pregnancy, age at menarche and menopause, and fertility treatments influence fibroid risk and growth can help inform preventive strategies, management approaches, and counseling for women affected by fibroids.

Lifestyle and Environmental Factors

Lifestyle and environmental factors, including diet and nutrition, obesity and physical activity, and environmental exposures, such as endocrine disruptors, can influence the

risk of developing uterine fibroids. How these factors relate to fibroid risk is as follows:
- *Diet and nutrition:*
  - *High-fat and high-calorie diets:* Diets high in fat and calories, particularly saturated fats and processed foods, have been associated with an increased risk of fibroids. These dietary patterns may contribute to obesity and hormonal imbalances, which can promote fibroid growth.
  - *Fruits and vegetables:* Conversely, diets rich in fruits, vegetables, and fiber have been associated with a reduced risk of fibroids. Antioxidants and phytochemicals found in fruits and vegetables may have protective effects against fibroids by reducing inflammation and oxidative stress.
  - *Red meat and dairy:* Some studies suggest that high consumption of red meat and dairy products may be associated with an increased risk of fibroids. These foods may contain hormones and growth factors that could influence fibroid growth.[3]
- *Obesity and physical activity:*
  - *Obesity:* It is a well-established risk factor for uterine fibroids. Excess body weight, particularly visceral fat, is associated with higher estrogen levels and insulin resistance, which can promote fibroid growth. Obese women are more likely to develop fibroids, have larger fibroids, and experience more severe symptoms compared to nonobese women.
  - *Physical activity:* Regular physical activity has been associated with a reduced risk of fibroids. Exercise may help maintain a healthy weight, improve insulin sensitivity, and reduce inflammation, all of which could contribute to a lower risk of fibroids. However, the specific effects of physical activity on fibroid risk require further investigation.
- *Environmental exposures (endocrine disruptors):*
  - *EDCs:* Exposure to EDCs, such as BPA, phthalates, and polychlorinated biphenyls (PCBs), has been implicated in the development of fibroids. EDCs can interfere with hormone signaling pathways, including estrogen and progesterone pathways, potentially promoting fibroid growth. These chemicals are commonly found in plastics, personal care products, pesticides, and industrial pollutants.
  - *Pesticides and herbicides:* Exposure to certain pesticides and herbicides, particularly organochlorine compounds, has been associated with an increased risk of fibroids. These chemicals may disrupt hormone balance and affect reproductive health.

MEDICAL CONDITIONS AND THERAPIES

Medical conditions and therapies can influence the risk of developing uterine fibroids and may impact their clinical course. How associations with conditions like hypertension and diabetes, as well as the influence of medications such as contraceptives and HRT, relate to fibroid risk is as follows:
- *Associations with conditions like hypertension and diabetes:*
  - *Hypertension (high blood pressure):* Hypertension has been associated with an increased risk of uterine fibroids. High blood pressure may affect blood flow to the uterus and promote the growth of fibroids. Additionally, hypertension is often

associated with obesity and metabolic syndrome, which are also risk factors for fibroids.
- *Diabetes:* Diabetes, particularly type 2 diabetes, has been linked to an increased risk of fibroids. Insulin resistance, a hallmark of type 2 diabetes, may contribute to fibroid growth by increasing insulin and insulin-like growth factor (IGF) levels, which can stimulate cell proliferation. Diabetes is also associated with obesity and hormonal imbalances, which are known risk factors for fibroids.

- *Influence of medications:*
  - *Contraceptives:* Hormonal contraceptives, including COCs containing estrogen and progestin, and progestin-only contraceptives (such as the progestin-releasing intrauterine device or depot medroxyprogesterone acetate injections), may influence the risk of fibroids. While COCs have been associated with a reduced risk of fibroids due to their suppressive effect on ovarian hormone production, progestin-only contraceptives may have variable effects on fibroid growth.
  - *HRT:* HRT, used to alleviate symptoms of menopause, typically involves ERT alone or in combination with progestin. While ERT may alleviate menopausal symptoms, it can also stimulate fibroid growth in some women. Adding progestin to ERT may help mitigate this risk by counteracting the proliferative effects of estrogen on fibroids.

- *Other medications and therapies:*
  - *Gonadotropin-releasing hormone (GnRH) agonists and antagonists:* These are medications used to temporarily shrink fibroids and relieve symptoms. These medications work by suppressing ovarian hormone production, leading to a temporary reduction in estrogen and progesterone levels. While effective in managing symptoms, their use is limited to the short term due to potential side effects and concerns about bone density loss.
  - *Nonsteroidal anti-inflammatory drugs (NSAIDs):* NSAIDs may be used to alleviate pain associated with fibroids. While NSAIDs do not directly influence fibroid growth, they can help relieve symptoms such as pelvic pain and discomfort.

CLINICAL IMPLICATIONS AND FUTURE DIRECTIONS

Impact on Health and Quality of Life

The presence of uterine fibroids can significantly impact health and quality of life, leading to various symptoms, complications, increased healthcare utilization, and economic burden. How uterine fibroids affect health and quality of life is as follows:

- *Symptoms and complications*: Uterine fibroids can cause a range of symptoms, including:
  - *Menstrual irregularities:* Heavy or prolonged menstrual bleeding (menorrhagia), irregular menstrual cycles, and breakthrough bleeding
  - *Pelvic pain and pressure:* Pelvic discomfort, pain during intercourse (dyspareunia), pelvic pressure, and lower back pain
  - *Urinary symptoms:* Frequent urination, urinary urgency, difficulty emptying the bladder, and urinary incontinence
  - *Reproductive issues:* Infertility, recurrent miscarriages, and complications during pregnancy and childbirth (e.g., preterm labor, breech presentation)

- Complications associated with uterine fibroids may include anemia due to heavy menstrual bleeding, urinary tract infections (UTIs) or urinary retention from bladder compression, and infertility or pregnancy complications due to fibroid-related changes in the uterus.
- *Healthcare utilization and economic burden:*
  - Uterine fibroids are a leading cause of gynecologic visits, accounting for significant healthcare utilization and costs. Women with fibroids may require frequent medical consultations, diagnostic tests (e.g., ultrasound, MRI), and treatments (e.g., medications, surgery) to manage their symptoms and complications.
  - The economic burden of uterine fibroids includes direct medical costs (e.g., healthcare services, medications, surgical procedures) as well as indirect costs (e.g., productivity losses, absenteeism from work, decreased quality of life). Fibroid-related healthcare costs can be substantial, particularly for women with severe symptoms or complications requiring surgical intervention.
- *Impact on quality of life:*
  - Uterine fibroids can have a profound impact on a woman's physical, emotional, and social well-being, affecting various aspects of daily life and functioning.
  - Chronic symptoms, such as pelvic pain, heavy menstrual bleeding, and urinary symptoms, can disrupt work, social activities, relationships, and overall quality of life.
  - Fibroid-related fertility issues and pregnancy complications may also cause significant emotional distress and anxiety for women and their partners.[7]

PREVENTION AND MANAGEMENT STRATEGIES[8,9]

Prevention and management strategies for uterine fibroids aim to alleviate symptoms, reduce fibroid size, prevent complications, and improve overall quality of life. These strategies encompass lifestyle modifications, pharmacological interventions, and various treatment options, including surgical and minimally invasive procedures. An overview of each approach is as follows:

- *Lifestyle modifications:*
  - *Healthy diet:* Adopting a balanced diet rich in fruits, vegetables, whole grains, and lean proteins can support overall health and may help reduce the risk of fibroids. Limiting intake of high-fat, high-calorie foods, processed foods, and red meat may be beneficial.
  - *Regular exercise:* Engaging in regular physical activity can help maintain a healthy weight, improve cardiovascular health, and reduce inflammation, which may have a positive impact on fibroid symptoms and overall well-being.
  - *Stress management:* Stress reduction techniques such as mindfulness meditation, yoga, deep breathing exercises, and relaxation therapies may help alleviate symptoms and improve coping mechanisms for women with fibroids.
- *Pharmacological interventions:*[8]
  - *Hormonal therapy:* Hormonal medications, including gonadotropin-releasing hormone (GnRH) agonists, progestins, and COCs, may be used to regulate menstrual bleeding, relieve

symptoms, and temporarily shrink fibroids.
- *NSAIDs:* NSAIDs such as ibuprofen or naproxen may help reduce pelvic pain, cramping, and discomfort associated with fibroids by reducing inflammation and inhibiting prostaglandin production.
- *Tranexamic acid:* This is a medication that can help reduce heavy menstrual bleeding associated with fibroids by promoting blood clotting and reducing blood loss during menstruation.
- *Surgical and minimally invasive treatments:*
  - *Myomectomy:* This is a surgical procedure to remove fibroids while preserving the uterus. It may be recommended for women who wish to preserve fertility or avoid hysterectomy.
  - *Hysterectomy:* This involves the surgical removal of the uterus and is considered a definitive treatment for uterine fibroids, particularly in women who have completed childbearing or have severe symptoms.
  - *Uterine artery embolization (UAE):* This is a minimally invasive procedure that involves blocking the blood supply to fibroids, leading to their shrinkage and symptom relief.
  - *MRI-guided focused ultrasound surgery (MRgFUS):* This is a noninvasive procedure that uses focused ultrasound energy to heat and destroy fibroid tissue while preserving surrounding structures.
- *Alternative and complementary therapies:*
  - *Acupuncture:* This may help alleviate fibroid-related symptoms such as pain and heavy bleeding, although research on its effectiveness is limited.
  - *Herbal remedies:* Certain herbal supplements, such as *Vitex* (chaste tree berry), green tea extract, and turmeric, have been studied for their potential benefits in managing fibroid symptoms, but the evidence is inconclusive.

RESEARCH CHALLENGES AND OPPORTUNITIES

Research in uterine fibroids faces several challenges and opportunities, particularly in the areas of epidemiological methods, integration of multi-omic data, and precision medicine approaches. A closer look at these aspects is given in the following text:

- *Advancements in epidemiological methods*:
  - *Challenge*: Despite being a common gynecological condition, uterine fibroids present challenges in epidemiological research due to their heterogeneity in terms of symptomatology, clinical presentation, and outcomes. Variability in fibroid size, location, growth rate, and response to treatment further complicates epidemiological studies.
  - *Opportunity*: Advances in epidemiological methods, including large-scale population-based studies, longitudinal cohort studies, and electronic health record (EHR)-based research, offer opportunities to better understand the natural history of fibroids, identify risk factors, and evaluate the effectiveness of preventive and treatment interventions. Collaborative efforts involving interdisciplinary teams and international consortia can facilitate data sharing and harmonization across studies, enabling more robust and generalizable findings.

- *Integration of multi-omic data:*
  - *Challenge:* Uterine fibroids are influenced by complex interactions between genetic, epigenetic, environmental, and hormonal factors. Traditional single-omic approaches may provide limited insights into the underlying mechanisms of fibroid pathogenesis and heterogeneity.
  - *Opportunity:* Integration of multi-omic data, including genomics, epigenomics, transcriptomics, proteomics, metabolomics, and microbiomics, offers a comprehensive view of fibroid biology and etiology. Systems biology approaches, such as network analysis and pathway modeling, can elucidate molecular pathways, identify key biomarkers, and uncover novel therapeutic targets. Longitudinal multi-omic studies can capture dynamic changes in gene expression, epigenetic regulation, and metabolic profiles over time, providing insights into disease progression and treatment response.
- *Precision medicine approaches:*
  - *Challenge:* Current treatments for uterine fibroids, such as hormonal therapies and surgical interventions, are often one-size-fits-all approaches that may not fully address individual variability in symptoms, treatment response, and outcomes. Precision medicine approaches tailored to the unique characteristics of each patient are needed to optimize treatment outcomes and minimize side effects.
  - *Opportunity:* Precision medicine approaches leverage patient-specific factors, including genetic variants, molecular profiles, clinical phenotypes, and lifestyle factors, to guide personalized treatment decisions. Stratification of patients based on molecular subtypes, biomarker profiles, and predictive algorithms can identify individuals who are most likely to benefit from specific interventions, enabling targeted therapies and individualized care plans. Integration of patient-reported outcomes, digital health technologies, and shared decision-making tools can further enhance patient engagement and satisfaction with care.

CONCLUSION

In conclusion, understanding the epidemiology and risk factors of uterine fibroids is essential for elucidating the burden of this prevalent gynecological condition and informing strategies for prevention, diagnosis, and management. Through epidemiological research, we have gained insights into the global prevalence rates, variation among different populations, incidence patterns, demographic patterns, and factors influencing fibroid risk.

Risk factors such as hormonal influences, genetic predisposition, reproductive factors, lifestyle and environmental factors, medical conditions, and therapies contribute to the complex etiology of fibroids. Genetic and epigenetic influences, hormonal regulation, and cellular and molecular mechanisms underlie the pathogenesis of fibroids, highlighting the multifactorial nature of this condition.

Challenges remain in conducting epidemiological studies due to the heterogeneity of fibroids and the need for advanced research methodologies. However, advancements in epidemiological methods, integration of multi-omic data, and precision medicine approaches offer promising avenues for furthering our understanding of fibroids and improving patient care.

REFERENCES

1. Baird DD, Dunson DB, Hill MC, Cousins D, Schectman JM. High cumulative incidence of uterine leiomyoma in black and white women: Ultrasound evidence. Am J Obstet Gynecol. 2003;188(1):100-7.
2. Wise LA, Palmer JR, Harlow BL, Spiegelman D, Stewart EA, Adams-Campbell LL, et al. Reproductive factors, hormonal contraception, and risk of uterine leiomyomata in African-American women: a prospective study. Am J Epidemiol. 2004;159(2):113-23.
3. Wise LA, Radin RG, Palmer JR, Kumanyika SK, Rosenberg L. A prospective study of dairy intake and risk of uterine leiomyomata. Am J Epidemiol. 2010;171(2):221-32.
4. Marshall LM, Spiegelman D, Barbieri RL, Goldman MB, Manson JE, Colditz GA, et al. Variation in the incidence of uterine leiomyoma among premenopausal women by age and race. Obstet Gynecol. 1997;90(6):967-73.
5. Ross RK, Pike MC, Vessey MP, Bull D, Yeates D, Casagrande JT. Risk factors for uterine fibroids: reduced risk associated with oral contraceptives. Br Med J (Clin Res Ed). 1986;293(6543):359-62.
6. Wise LA, Laughlin-Tommaso SK. Epidemiology of uterine fibroids: from menarche to menopause. Clin Obstet Gynecol. 2016;59(1):2-24.
7. Islam MS, Protic O, Giannubilo SR, Toti P, Tranquilli AL, Petraglia F, et al. Uterine leiomyoma: available medical treatments and new possible therapeutic options. J Clin Endocrinol Metab. 2013;98(3):921-34.
8. Stewart EA, Nicholson WK, Bradley L, Borah BJ. The burden of uterine fibroids for African-American women: results of a national survey. J Womens Health (Larchmt). 2013;22(10):807-16.
9. Marsh EE, Al-Hendy A, Kappus D, Galitsky A, Stewart EA, Kerolous M. Burden, Prevalence, and treatment of uterine fibroids: a survey of U.S. women. J Womens Health (Larchmt). 2018;27(11):1359-67.

CHAPTER 2

Classification of Fibroid Uterus

Sharmin Abbasi, Neharika Malhotra, Mohammad Noor A Alam

■ INTRODUCTION

The fibroid uterus is one of the most common benign gynecological tumors in the reproductive age of a woman. Fibroid uteri arise from the monoclonal smooth muscle of myometrium. They are the benign tumor and their growth depends on hormonal stimulation, especially estrogen and progesterone.[1] Fibroids may enlarge during pregnancy or those who are taking oral contraceptives. They may regress with the menopausal phase of life. The pathogenesis of fibroids is poorly understood.

Most women with fibroid are asymptomatic and some patients have symptoms which vary according to the classification of fibroid. Fibroids can either be diagnosed as asymptomatic with imaging findings or be symptomatic.[2] The common symptoms are menorrhagia, pelvic pain, and pressure symptoms to surrounding organs. Symptoms of fibroids vary according to their different location. For the diagnosis, physical examination and imaging are helpful.[3] Correct classification of fibroid is important for the planning of treatment and prevention of further complications.

Treatment ranges from expectant management to surgical treatment. Uterine fibroids contribute to one-third to half of all hysterectomies globally. Some patients may present with complications of fibroids. Very rarely it turns to malignancy (<1%). At the same time, its high prevalence affects the economic burden on the healthcare system.[4] In addition to direct economic burden, it also puts indirect effects by absence from work or disability.[5]

■ EPIDEMIOLOGY

There are large numbers of fibroids which remain undetected which makes a significant bias in epidemiological data. The prevalence of fibroid varies from 5% to 80% according to the diagnostic methods and ethnic variations of the study population.[6] Fibroids are present during the reproductive age. They are rare before puberty and in late menopause. Some risk factors are associated with fibroids including old age, nulliparity, obesity, early menarche, vitamin D deficiency, altered microbiota, obesity, excessive vitamin E level, intrauterine exposure to diethylstilbestrol (DES), early age exposure to isoflavones, and relaxer of hair. Exposure to endocrine-disrupting chemicals, especially organophosphate esters and plasticizers, and family history of fibroid in first-degree relatives are also risk factors. The global variations of the burden of uterine fibroids are pivotal.[7] Fibroid incidence is two- to three-fold more in Black and Asian Chinese women than white women.

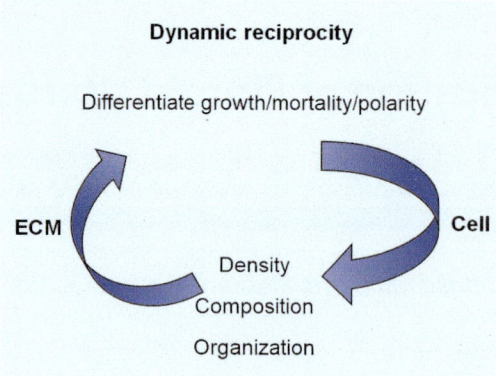

Fig. 1: Extracellular matrix (ECM) and uterine fibroid related to the pathophysiology of fibroid uterus.

■ PATHOPHYSIOLOGY

The pathophysiology of uterine fibroid is poorly understood. Inappropriate growth of smooth muscle of the uterus, DNA damage, growth factor, transforming growth factor beta, and extracellular matrix remodeling are connected with the pathophysiology process (Fig. 1).

■ EVALUATION

History and physical examination including proper menstrual history are helpful for proper evaluation. Common presenting symptoms are menorrhagia and metrorrhagia. Pelvic pain, dyspareunia, bowel symptoms, urinary problems, and anemia should be kept in mind. Prevaginal examination which includes per speculum and bimanual examination is done to exclude any cervical and vaginal pathology.

■ DIAGNOSTIC TOOLS

Transvaginal ultrasonography (TVS) is very helpful for imaging of uterine fibroids. Saline infusion sonography (SIS) will give more additional information with TVS, especially to find out subserous and intramural fibroid. A well-circumscribed, hypoechoic mass will appear in sonography findings. Calcification and necrosis distort echogenicity.[8]

Hysterosalpingography (HSG) is helpful for the diagnosis of fibroid but nowadays, it is not widely used.[9]

Magnetic resonance imaging (MRI) is superior because it gives more accurate findings of fibroids regarding size, blood supply, margin, and location related to other pelvic organs. For the proper classification of fibroid, MRI is very helpful.[10]

Hysteroscopy will help to see the interior of the uterus. This imaging helps to visualize the location of the fibroid inside the cavity. Using this procedure, "see and treat" approaches allow to remove the intrauterine fibroids.[11]

■ CLASSIFICATION OF FIBROID

There are various classification systems. They are described in the following text.

Classification by Anatomical Location (Figs. 2A and B; Flowchart 1)

- *Fibroid in the body of the uterus*: Most of the fibroids are in the body of the uterus and they are usually multiple in number. In the body of the uterus, they are divided into the following:
  - *Interstitial or intramural (70–75%)*: This is the most common type of fibroid. In the wall of the uterus between the fibers of muscle, most intramural fibroids will grow. They are intramural in position and eventually, they are pushed to outer or inner directions.

    They are classified according to their location of growth:
    - *Anterior intramural fibroid:* Located on the anterior wall of the uterus

Classification of Fibroid Uterus

Types of uterine fibroids

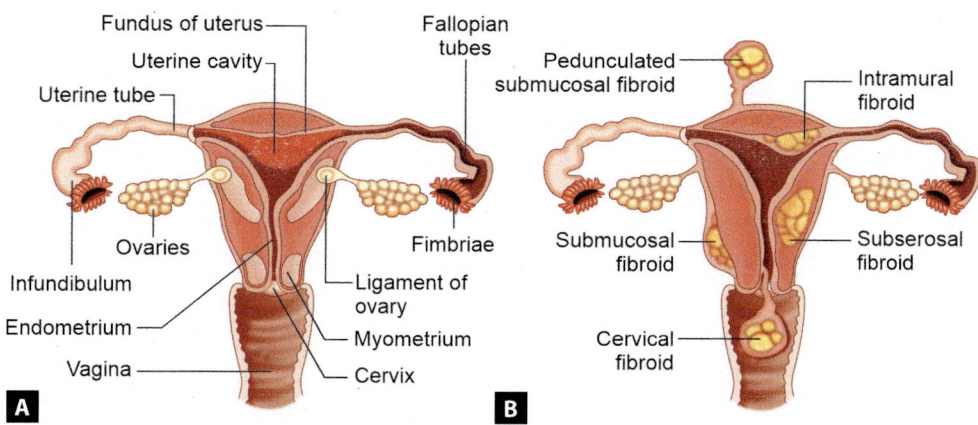

Figs. 2A and B: Anatomical distributions of fibroid uterus.

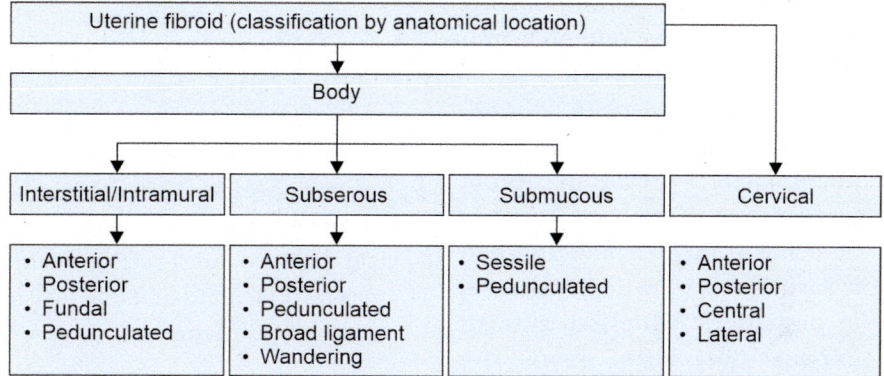

- *Posterior intramural fibroid:* Located on the posterior wall of the uterus
- *Fundal intramural fibroid:* Located on the top or fundal part of the uterus
- *Pedunculated:* When they are attached by a stalk or peduncle inside of the uterus
- *Subperitoneal or subserous (8–10%):* When the fibroid grows on the outside of the uterus and below the serosa or smooth outer layer, it is called subserous. Its growth can be on the uterine tissue or it can be attached by a stalk. Due to its location, this fibroid can push against the pelvis and closer organs. It is located outside of the uterus and is less likely to cause abnormal uterine bleeding. Subserous fibroids mostly cause pressure symptoms to surrounding organs.

Depending on the location of subserous fibroids, they are classified into the following:
- *Anterior subserous fibroid:* It is located on the anterior side of the uterus and may give pressure

symptoms on the urinary bladder and is associated with urinary symptoms.
- *Posterior subserous fibroid:* It is located on the posterior side of the uterus. When it becomes large, then it presses the bowel or sciatic nerve. As pressure symptoms, it causes constipation, pain in leg, or lower back pain.
- *Pedunculated subserous fibroid:* When the fibroid is attached to the uterine wall by a stalk or peduncle in the outer side of the uterus, it is called pedunculated fibroid. Intense cramp-like pain and excessive bleeding during menstruation are common symptoms of this type of fibroid.
- *Wandering or parasitic fibroid:* This fibroid is a rare type. When the pedunculated subserous fibroid undergoes torsion, gets torn, or detaches from the pedicle, then it sustains its growth by omental or mesenteric adhesion through neovascularization from the surrounding tissues. It may also develop by de novo after peritoneal metaplasia (diffuse peritoneal leiomyomatosis) or after surgery and morcellation procedures.
- *Broad ligament or pseudofibroid:* When the subserous or pedunculated fibroid extends into the peritoneal folds of broad ligament, then it is called broad ligament or intraligamentary fibroid. It has both clinical and surgical importance. It may cause pressure symptoms to the ureter and cause ureteric obstructions or hydroureter. During surgery injury to the ureter, uterine artery and concealed hematoma formation are the complications. During the examination, it may be confused with ovarian tumor. It causes pseudo-Meig syndrome.
- *Submucous fibroid (3–5%)*: When the fibroid is pushed toward the uterine cavity and presented beneath the endometrium, it is called a submucous fibroid. It usually distorts the uterine cavity. It causes maximum symptoms of abnormal uterine bleeding.

There are different types of submucous fibroids:
- *Pedunculated fibroids (polyp):* They are attached to the uterus by a stalk.
  - They may come out through cervix.
- *Sessile fibroids:* Fibroids without steam are called sessile.
■ *Cervical fibroid:* This is a rare variety of fibroid uterus (1–3%). When it grows, it will displace the cervix or the external os may be difficult to find out. It also disturbs the anatomy of the ureter.

In the supervaginal part, it may be divided into:
- Interstitial
- Subperitoneal
- Polypoidal

Depending upon the position it will be classified as follows:
- *Anterior:* They are placed in the anterior part of the cervix.
- *Posterior:* They are in the posterior part of the cervix.
- *Central:* They are in the mid-part of the cervix.
- *Lateral:* They are in the lateral or side portion of the cervix.

FIGO Classification System of Fibroid (Fig. 3)

The FIGO (International Federation of Gynaecology and Obstetrics) classification system was developed to maintain the uniformity of the classification of fibroid uterus with the help of clinical care and research works. Proper classification will help the clinicians to select the best management plan, post-treatment response and recurrence of disease.[10] The FIGO classification system of fibroids as follows:

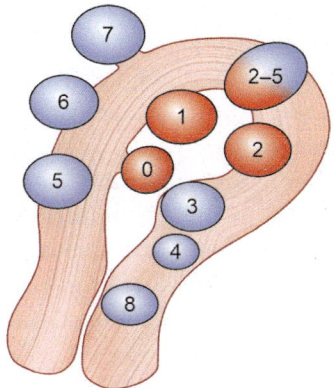

Fig. 3: FIGO classification system of fibroid uterus.

SM (sub-mucosal)	0	Pedunculated intracavitary
	1	<50% intramural (≥50% submucosal)
	2	≥50% intramural (<50% submucosal)
O (other)	3	100% intramural, contacting endometrium
	4	100% intramural, no endometrial or subserosal contact
	5	Subserosal, ≥50% intramural
	6	Subserosal, <50% intramural
	7	Pedunculated subserosal
	8	Nonmyometrial location: e.g., cervical, broad ligament, parasitic
Hybrid	x–x	Both submucosal and subserosal components. The first number designates the submucosal component and the second number designates the subserosal component
	2–5	Submucosal and subserosal each with less than half the diameter in the endometrial and peritoneal cavities, respectively

- *Submucosal fibroid: FIGO classification 0–2*
  Submucosa fibroids are located beneath the mucosal layer. They are classified according to their intramural extension. Pedunculated fibroids in group 0 are attached to the endometrium by connecting vascular stalk. Clinically, this group has significance because they are associated with most of clinical symptoms, such as menorrhagia, dysmenorrhea, infertility, and recurrent pregnancy loss. Hysteroscopic resection is more frequent management of these groups of fibroids.
- *Other: FIGO classification 3–8*
  Fibroids which do not contain the submucosal component are classified as other. These groups include intramural and subserous fibroids which contact the endometrium but do not extend to the endometrial cavity. For the diagnosis of FIGO 4, "claw sign" of the surrounding myometrium is an important finding on cross-sectional imaging. Subserosal fibroids according to their intramural extension are classified as FIGO 5, 6, 7. In FIGO 7 group, fibroids have pedunculated vascular stalk. Extrauterine fibroids are classified as FIGO 8 group. Clinically, they give pressure symptoms to adjacent structures, especially urinary bladder and colon. Treatment options include uterine

artery embolization, myomectomy, or hysterectomy.

- *Hybrid fibroid:* When the fibroid extends from the submucosa to the serosa, it is called a hybrid type. It is expressed as a number. The first number is the relation of fibroid to the endometrium and the second number to the serosa. Treatment options are uterine artery embolization, MRI-guided focused ultrasound (MRg-FUS).

Limitations of the FIGO Classification System

Interpretation variability has been seen between gynecologists and radiologists. If misclassification occurs, then it may lead to improper surgical planning. If the size and number of fibroids will increase, it causes distortion of uterine demarcation and the classifications become more discrepant among clinicians.

Classification According to the Stiffness and Rigidity of Fibroid

The stiffness and rigidity are measured by special ultrasonography which is called shear wave elastography (SWE). SWE makes acoustic radiofrequency impulse which is transversely oriented through the surrounding tissues. TVS and SWE together comprise a new imaging tool for the classification according to the stiffness of the tissue. It is proposed by the University of Chicago **(Fig. 4)**.

Proposed classification system according to rigidity based on SWE.

Composite SWE score/uterus
- *AL1:* Soft fibroid
- *AL2:* Pliable fibroid
- *AL3:* Firm fibroid
- *AL4:* Hard fibroid

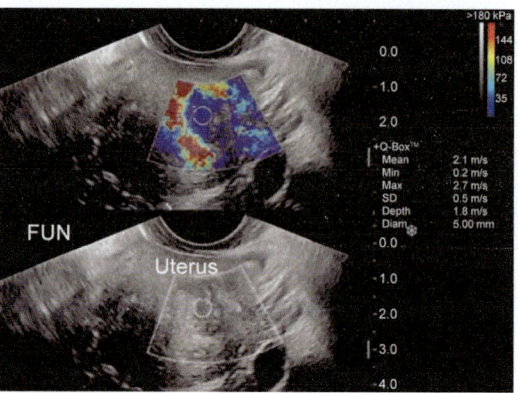

Fig. 4: Strain ratio elastography findings of fibroid uterus. (FUN: fundus)

TABLE 1: Wamsteker classification of submucous fibroid.

Type	Feature
Type 0	- Entirely within endometrial cavity - No myometrial extension
Type I	- <50% myometrial extension - <90° angle of myoma surface to uterine wall
Type II	- >50% myometrial extension - >90° angle of myoma surface to uterine wall

Source: Adopted by European Society for Gynecological Endoscopy (ESGE) and FIGO classification system of fibroid.

Wamsteker Classification of Submucous Fibroid

Wamsteker classification is done depending on the degree of penetration of fibroid to myometrium and angle of fibroid with the uterine cavity **(Table 1 and Fig. 5)**.

STEP-W or Lasmar Classification of Fibroid Uterus

In 2005, hysteroscopic myoma classification, the "STEP-W or Lasmar" classification,

Classification of Fibroid Uterus

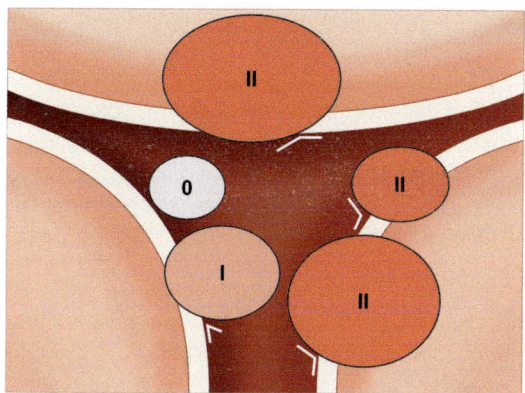

Fig. 5: Wamsteker classification of submucous fibroid.

was established. This is a preoperative classification of myoma which evaluates the viability and degree of difficulty of hysteroscopic myomectomy **(Tables 2 and 3 and Fig. 6)**.[11]

MUSA Consensus

MUSA (Morphological Uterus Sonographic Assessment) is formulated to use systemic steps to assess and report ultrasound findings of myometrium and associated fibroids **(Table 4)**.

TABLE 2: STEP-W or Lasmar classification of fibroid uterus.

	Size (cm)	Topography	Extension of the base	Penetration	Lateral wall	Total
0	<2	Low	<1/3	0	+1	
1	2–5	Middle	1/3–2/3	<50%		
2	>5	Upper	>2/3	>50%		

TABLE 3: STEP-W submucous fibroid classification.

Score	Group	Complexity and therapeutic
0–4	I	• Low complexity • Hysteroscopic myomectomy
5–6	II	• High complexity • Hysteroscopic myomectomy • Consider GnRH use • Consider two steps • Hysteroscopic myomectomy
7–8	III	Consider alternative to hysteroscopy

(GnRH: gonadotropin-releasing hormone)

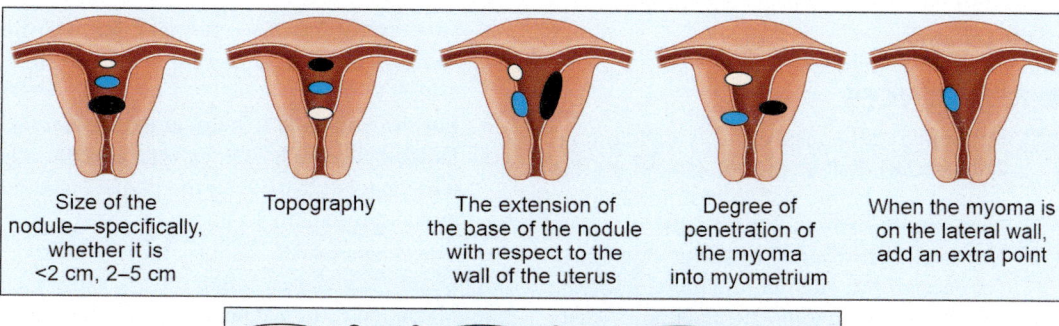

Fig. 6: STEP-W or Lasmar classification of fibroid uterus.

Parameter	Criteria
TABLE 4: MUSA Consensus.	
Uterus	Measure the length, A–P diameter, transverse diameter, volume
Serosal contour	Regular or lobulated
Wall of myometrium	Symmetrical or asymmetrical
Myometrial echogenicity	Homogeneous or heterogeneous
Myometrial lesions	*Margin:* Well defined or ill defined
	Number of lesions
	Site: Anterior, posterior, fundal, right/left lateral, global
	Type: According to FIGO classification
	Size: Three perpendicular diameters
	Outer lesion-free margin: Distance from the serosal surface
	Inner lesion-free margin: Distance from the endometrial surface
	Echogenicity: Hypoechoic, isoechoic, or hyperechoic

(A–P: anteroposterior; FIGO: International Federation of Gynaecology and Obstetrics; MUSA: Morphological Uterus Sonographic Assessment)

CONCLUSION

The structured, illustrated classification of fibroids will help to formulate a proper diagnosis, counseling of the patient, and at the same time facilitate selecting the highest appropriate medical and surgical treatment plan for the patient. A gynecologist should follow the proper classification system to avoid possible complications and treatment failure. Implementation of the proper classification system of fibroid can reduce misdiagnosis and will improve the outcome of the patients.

REFERENCES

1. Deshmukh SP, Gonsalves CF, Guglielmo FF, Mitchell DG. Role of MR imaging of uterine leiomyomas before and after embolization. Radiographic. 2012;32(6):E251-81.
2. Day Baird D, Dunson DB, Hill MC, Cousins D, Schectman JM. High cumulative incidence of uterine leiomyoma in black and white women: ultrasound evidence. Am J Obstet Gynecol. 2003;188(1):100-7.
3. Hossain MZ, Rahman MM, Ullah MM, Mukthadira M, Akter FA, Jahan AB, et al. A comparative study of magnetic resonance imaging and transabdominal ultrasonography for the diagnosis and evaluation of uterine fibroids. Mymensingh Med J. 2017;26(4):821-7.
4. Donnez J, Dolmans MM. Uterine fbroid management: from the present to the future. Hum Reprod Update. 2016;22(6):665-86.
5. Abdullah B, Subramaniam R, Omar S, Wragg P, Ramli N, Wui A, et al. Magnetic resonance-guided focused ultrasound surgery (MRgFUS) treatment for uterine fibroids. Biomed Imaging Interv J. 2010; 6(2):e15.
6. Puri K, Famuyide AO, Erwin PJ, Stewart EA, Laughlin-Tommaso SK. Submucosal fibroids and the relation to heavy menstrual bleeding and anemia. Am J Obstet Gynecol. 2014; 210(1):38. e1-38. e387.
7. Shalev J, Meizner I, Bar-Hava I, Dicker D, Mashiach R, Ben-Rafael Z. Predictive value of transvaginal sonography performed before routine diagnostic hysteroscopy

for evaluation of infertility. Fertil Steril. 2000;73(2):412-7.
8. Stewart EA. Clinical practice. Uterine fibroids. N Engl J Med. 2015;372(17):1646-55.
9. Ahmadi F, Zafarani F, Niknejadi M, Vosough A. Uterine leiomyoma: hysterosalpingographic appearances. Int J Fertil Steril. 2007; 1:137-44.
10. Gomez E, Nguyen MLT, Fursevich D, Macura K, Gupta A. MRI-based pictorial review of the FIGO classification system for uterine fibroids. Abdom Radiol (NY). 2021;46:2146-55.
11. Piecak K, Milart P. Hysteroscopic myomectomy. Przegląd Menopauzalny. 2017; 16:126-8.

CHAPTER 3

Ultrasound Assessment and Differential Diagnosis of Uterine Fibroids

Aruna Nigam, Asma Khanday, Subohi Khan, Shivangini Varshney

■ INTRODUCTION

Uterine fibroids are one of the most common benign tumors in reproductive age-group females that may or may not be symptomatic. The most common modality for the diagnosis is ultrasonography (USG). USG is very specific and sensitive and can guide regarding the treatment in the majority of the cases.

Uterine fibroids/leiomyomas are estrogen sensitive and generally regress during menopause. The most common diagnostic modality is USG, and very commonly asymptomatic fibroids are reported incidentally on ultrasound performed for nongynecological problems. Although USG is highly specific and sensitive, it depends on operator skill and machine quality.

Ultrasonography as the first-line imaging modality for fibroid can be done transvaginally or transabdominally. It can also be combined with a Doppler to assess vascularity, differentiate from other tumors, and evaluate the adnexa. Saline infusion sonography (SIS) can also be done to assess the submucous fibroid and distinguish it from an endometrial polyp. Three-dimensional (3D) ultrasound can be done to do the fibroid mapping before surgery.

In the following sections, various aspects of the use of USG for the diagnosis of fibroid uterus have been discussed in detail.

■ APPEARANCE OF LEIOMYOMAS IN SONOGRAPHY

In general, uterine leiomyomas appear as well-defined, solid, concentric, hypoechoic lesions **(Fig. 1)**. Echogenicity may differ depending on the amount of calcification and fibrous tissue. They may cause variable degrees of acoustic shadowing. Calcification may appear as echogenic foci with acoustic shadowing.[1] In cases of necrosis and degeneration, the area may appear as anechoic in the myoma. Small myomas are difficult to locate and may just appear as irregularity/bulge in the myometrial wall. Lower segment myoma may compress the cervical canal leading to fluid collection in the uterine cavity. This is especially prominent

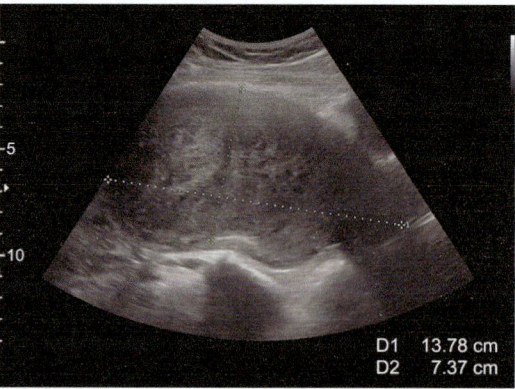

Fig. 1: Ultrasound image of a large intramural fibroid with subserosal component seen in the anterior uterine wall (FIGO 5).

during menstruation and also helps in delineation. Any leiomyoma may undergo internal hemorrhage, fibrosis, calcification, atrophy, or several types of degeneration.

Important parameters that need to be assessed during the USG examination are as follows:

- *Location:* This needs to be seen to classify the type of leiomyoma as per FIGO-AUB (International Federation of Gynecology and Obstetrics-abnormal uterine bleeding) classification of leiomyomas[2] as discussed in the previous chapter. Fundal myomas are generally asymptomatic unless they displace the endometrium. They may cause pressure symptoms. Myomas on the posterior myometrium need to be differentiated from adenomyomas as the latter are mostly located in the posterior myometrium. Whenever seeing the lower segment fibroid **(Fig. 2)**, one must evaluate the ureters and kidney for hydroureter and hydronephrosis. Leiomyomas may also appear outside the uterus such as round ligament, cervix, vagina, or over intestinal wall in case of parasitic fibroid. Adding MRI in these conditions helps delineate the exact characteristics.

Lasmar/STEP-W[3] classification is also based on the USG findings preoperatively for submucous myomas. The classification was developed to evaluate the viability and the degree of difficulty of hysteroscopic myomectomy as discussed in the previous chapter. The STEP-W classification takes into account not only the degree of penetration of the myoma into the myometrium but also parameters like the distance of the base of the myoma from the uterine wall, the size of the nodule (cm), and the topography of the uterine cavity.

- *Size and number:* Along with site, the size and number of fibroids are very important to classify them into various types and also surgically for doing fibroid mapping. This helps in deciding the incision preoperatively and the idea regarding enucleation with the minimum number of incisions to avoid adhesions. This also helps in counseling of the patient regarding recurrence in case of myomectomy.
- *Distance and displacement of endometrium* **(Fig. 3)**: Again, this is important when differentiating between type 3 (touching endometrium) and type 4 myomas. Patient's symptoms can also be correlated as myomas displacing endometrium are symptomatic. These myomas also create problems during embryo transfer because of the difficult insertion of catheters (especially the lower segment fibroids). Mention of distance from the endometrium will also help during surgery to make one careful during dissection and saving the entry in the endometrial cavity.

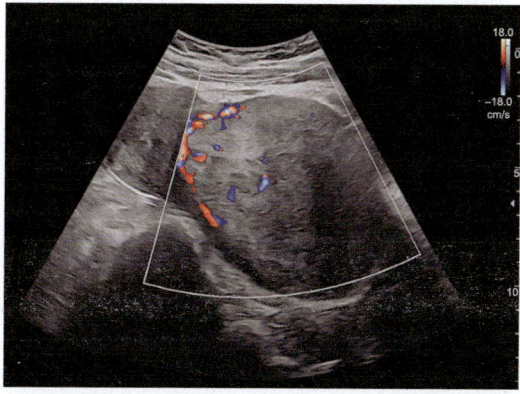

Fig. 2: Ultrasound images of a large hybrid fibroid as seen in the anterior myometrium involving the uterocervical region (FIGO 2–5) and also showing peripheral vascularization with multiple feeding vessels.

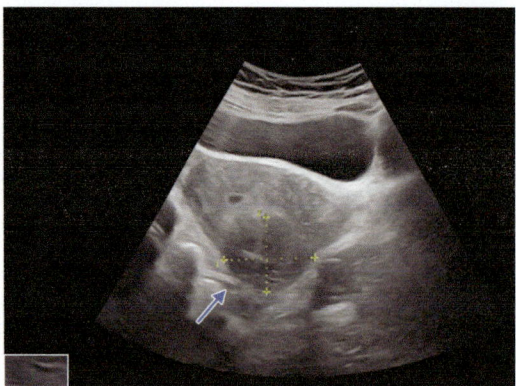

Fig. 3: Uterus appears bulky and shows a well-defined heterogeneously hypoechoic lesion in the posterior myometrium measuring ~4.5 × 3.6 cm and displacing the endometrium anteriorly, suggestive of a posterior intramural fibroid.

- *Relationship with other organs:* Besides compression of the urinary tract, large fibroids may compress on the intestine causing decreased appetite or constipation. Broad ligament or cornual fibroids will stretch the fallopian tube leading to infertility.
- *Vascularity:* Addition of Doppler flow during ultrasound imaging to fibroids shows circumferential vascularity **(Fig. 2)**. No vascularity is found in necrotic and degenerated myoma or in cases of myoma torsion.
- *Features of degeneration:* Degenerated fibroids may have different and varied echogenicity that need to be mentioned during USG examination as cystic degeneration will pose a challenge during surgery and red degeneration does not need any intervention.
- *Specific parameters during pregnancy:* All the above parameters are very important during pregnancy with special mention of location due to the following reasons:
  - Lower segment fibroid/cervical fibroid may lead to delayed engagement of the head or obstructed labor.
  - Lower segment fibroid may come at the incision site making cesarean section challenging.
  - Fibroids may lead to incoordinate uterine action.
  - Fibroids may cause postpartum hemorrhage, so one needs to be careful in the peripartum period.
  - If one decides on cesarean myomectomy, the idea of the location, site, and size will help in deciding upon the procedure.

■ TRANSVAGINAL SONOGRAPHY

In general, transvaginal sonography (TVS) is superior to transabdominal sonography (TAS) and most of the gynecologists are well versed in the intricacies of TVS in their practice. As the probe is closer to the uterus, it is especially helpful in detecting small leiomyomas, especially in the retroflexed and retroverted uterus. Three most important conditions where TVS has an added advantage are:
1. Obese women
2. *Women with excessive bowel gases:* In constipation
3. Women with the inability to hold urine for a long.

As TVS probes are of high frequency and short focal lengths, they have shallow depth of scan leading to problems in the scan in cases of:
- Large and fundal myomas
- Pedunculated myomas.

■ 3D ULTRASONOGRAPHY[4] (FIG. 4)

Three-dimensional USG is one of the latest developed techniques and is available with both transabdominal and transvaginal scans. It exhibits a multiplanar display of uterine anatomy. The uterus is shown in the standard orientation and in the coronal, transverse, and sagittal planes. Here, the operator is required

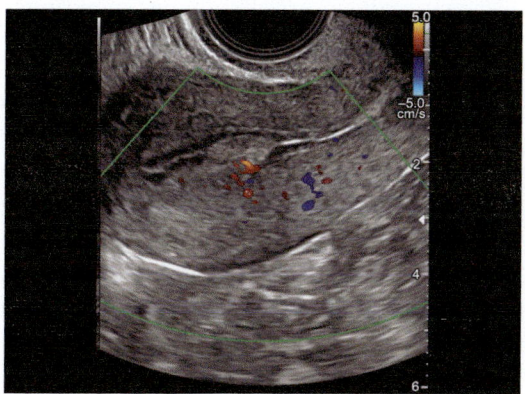

Fig. 4: Endometrial polyp: Round echogenic soft tissue within the endometrium with a vascular stalk posteriorly.

to rotate the volume to see the standard plane [i.e., transverse, sagittal, and coronal (C-plane)]. The display differs, depending on equipment and operator preference. The sagittal acquisition is normally superior to the coronal acquisition. If the uterus is massive to get into one volume with the sagittal plane, the transverse plane can be used. 3D TVS is generally better than 3D TAS. This is very helpful in assessing myoma volume and vascularity using the vascularity index or vascularity volume display. In addition to the multiplanar mode, the volume data may be also used for a multislice mode, rendered display mode, thick slice mode, or other modes (e.g., invert mode). In patients with a distorted endometrium, 3D USG may readily help in differentiating submucous myomas or endometrial polyps. It is now the first choice for the detection of Müllerian anomalies. This can also be helpful in fibroid mapping before surgery.

SALINE INFUSION SONOGRAPHY

Saline infusion sonohysterography (SIS) is a radiological imaging method utilized for scanning various endocervical and endometrial lesions. Using the same principles as ultrasound, this method visualizes the endometrial cavity which is predistended with saline. This is also very helpful in differentiating endometrial polyps with submucous fibroids.

DIFFERENTIAL DIAGNOSIS OF FIBROID DURING ULTRASONOGRAPHY

During ultrasonographic evaluation, it is very important to differentiate leiomyoma from adenomyosis/adenomyoma, solid adnexal masses, endometrial polyp, leiomyosarcoma, etc.

Adenomyosis/adenomyoma: This is a very important differential as the treatment/surgery of adenomyosis is more challenging and preoperative diagnosis helps in planning the surgical technique. For adenomyosis, MUSA (Morphological Uterus Sonographic Assessment) criteria[5] have been given by a radiologist which include globular uterine enlargement without the presence of leiomyomata, cystic anechoic spaces or lakes in the myometrium, subendometrial echoic linear striations, uterine wall thickening, heterogeneous echo texture, obscured endometrial/myometrial border, and thickening of the transition zone.

Adnexal pathologies can also be confused with subserosal fibroids, especially solid ovarian tumors, that is, Brenner, fibrothecomas. This especially occurs when subserosal fibroid is mainly extrauterine or pedunculated. Doppler sonography may help in these cases.

Submucosal fibroids and endometrial polyps are important to be differentiated **(Fig. 5)**. Polyps are homogenous hyperechoic, whereas echogenicity of submucous fibroid may vary depending on the nature

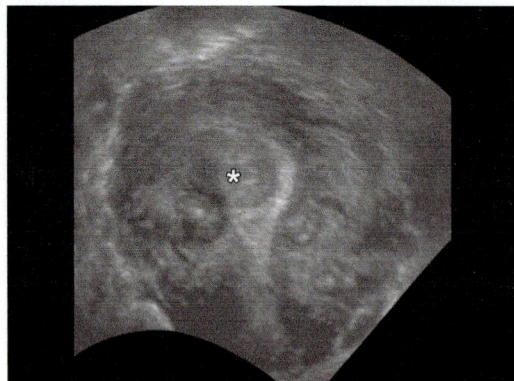

Fig. 5: C-plane image of the uterus with a submucosal fibroid.

and size. Polyps have generally single-feeder vessels with small bases, whereas submucous fibroids have multiple feeding vessels, larger bases, and extensions inside the myometrium. The endometrium lining gets splayed in the presence of polyp, whereas it is generally deviated in the case of fibroid. Saline sonography may help in delineation of the base in these cases. Adding 3D to the evaluation gives a very good evaluation. Strain elastography may supplement USG to visualize the different stiffness of endometrial polyps and submucosal leiomyomas.

Leiomyosarcoma: Another important but rare entity that needs to be differentiated is leiomyosarcoma as the treatment is different in this condition, and complete removal along with bilateral salpingo-oophorectomy is needed in this with cautionary note on no morcellation. There is no pelvic imaging technique that can reliably differentiate between them because both of them may show mixed echogenic and poor echogenic parts, central necrosis, color Doppler findings of irregular vessel distribution, low impedance to flow, and high peak systolic velocity. Here, MRI may be helpful.

Lipoleiomyomas

Lipoleiomyomas are rare fat-containing fibroids, with a reported prevalence of between 0.005% and 2%. They are nonmalignant and present with the same symptoms as uterine fibroids. The most common cause is thought to be fatty metamorphosis of the smooth muscle cells of leiomyoma. If pedunculated, they can be erroneously diagnosed on imaging as ovarian dermoids. At USG, they are typically echogenic masses, in contrast to the usually hypoechoic fibroids. On MRI, these tumors show high signals on both T1W and T2W images; often, they have a hypoechoic rim, which is thought to be due to a surrounding layer of the myometrium. A fat-suppression technique is useful to confirm the presence of fat.

Transient Myometrial Contractions

Myometrial contractions can be mistaken for uterine fibroids. However, the contractions are transient, and therefore the masses will disappear on subsequent scans.

■ CONCLUSION

- USG is the most common modality for the diagnosis of uterine fibroids.
- One must describe the site, size, number, and relationship with endometrium and nearby organs to classify the fibroid and decide upon the treatment.
- Adding 3D to USG can help a lot in fibroid mapping before surgery.
- Important entities that need to be differentiated are adenomyoma, solid adnexal masses, endometrial polyp, and leiomyosarcoma.

■ REFERENCES

1. Woźniak A, Woźniak S. Ultrasonography of uterine leiomyomas. Prz Menopauzalny. 2017;16(4):113-7.

2. Munro MG, Critchley HOD, Fraser IS; FIGO Menstrual Disorders Committee. The two FIGO systems for normal and abnormal uterine bleeding symptoms and classification of causes of abnormal uterine bleeding in the reproductive years: 2018 revisions. Int J Gynaecol Obstet. 2018;143(3):393-408.
3. Lasmar RB, Xinmei Z, Indman PD, Celeste RK, Di Spiezio Sardo A. Feasibility of a new system of classification of submucous myomas: a multicenter study. Fertil Steril. 2011;95(6):2073-7.
4. Ong CL. The current status of three-dimensional ultrasonography in gynaecology. Ultrasonography. 2016;35(1):13-24.
5. Van den Bosch T, Dueholm M, Leone FP, Valentin L, Rasmussen CK, Votino A, et al. Terms, definitions and measurements to describe sonographic features of myometrium and uterine masses: a consensus opinion from the morphological uterus sonographic assessment (MUSA) group. Ultrasound Obstet Gynecol. 2015;46: 284-98.

CHAPTER 4

Fibroids and Subfertility

Anshu Jindal

■ INTRODUCTION

Fibroids are the most common benign tumors in women of reproductive age group 21–45 years (30–40%).[1] Cavity-distorting fibroids could be the sole cause of subfertility in 2–3% of cases or they may be associated with other causes of infertility where their contribution to infertility is difficult to define.[2,3] Fibroids can vary in size, location, and clinical symptoms. Most of them are asymptomatic and hence may go unnoticed. Submucosal and intramural fibroids that distort the endometrial cavity are associated with lower pregnancy rates, implantation, and delivery rates in women undergoing assisted reproductive technology (ART) compared to infertile women without fibroids.[4]

■ HOW FIBROIDS IMPACT FERTILITY

The exact reason how fibroids affect fertility is not fully understood. However, various reasons have been cited to explain the reduced fertility, including increased uterine contractility, deranged cytokine profile, abnormal vascularization, chronic inflammation, and problems with sperm transport. Fibroids impact fertility by altering the endometrial receptivity (ER). *HOXA/HOXA 10* gene is an intrinsic component of implantation, decidualization, and immune modulation in the uterus.[5] Glycodelin A—a secretory glycoprotein—is abundant in the endometrium at the time of implantation enhancing angiogenesis and suppressing natural killer cell activity. The expression of both *HOXA 10* gene and glycodelin A is reduced with fibroids contributing to implantation failure. Uterine natural killer (uNK) cells and macrophages abundant at the time of implantation may be increased with fibroids impacting ER.[6] Fibroids nearer to the endometrial cavity affect the endometrial milieu making it unfavorable for implantation.

Thickening of the junctional zone and increased myometrial peristalsis as observed on cine-mode magnetic resonance imaging (MRI) is seen especially with cavity-distorting fibroids in the mid-luteal phase. This can contribute to implantation failure and early pregnancy losses.[7,8]

Leiomyomas have a pseudocapsule (PC) which is rich in neurotransmitters and markers of neovascularization, namely Endoglin and CD34.[9] Submucosal fibroids and cervical fibroids are endowed with a thicker PC, hence making the uterus more prone to abnormal uterine contractions.

Cavity-distorting leiomyomas secrete inflammatory vasoactive factors like transforming growth factor-beta (TGF-β) contributing to subfertility by making the endometrial environment unfavorable for implantation. This has been confirmed by several investigations.[10]

CAUSE OF FIBROIDS

Why fibroids form is largely unknown. Various genetic and epigenetic factors have been implicated in their causation. Fibroids seem to run in families as well as in certain races. Black women are three times more prone to developing fibroids 3 years earlier than White women. In addition, environmental factors, such as obesity, vitamin D deficiency, a diet rich in animal fats, refined carbohydrates, dairy products, high salt, and low-fiber diet, can contribute to their causation.[11,12]

The growth of fibroids seems to be positively associated with prolonged estrogen exposure. Hence, early menarche, late menopause, and obesity show a positive correlation with their growth. This is evident during pregnancy when the growth of fibroids may be enhanced under the influence of estrogens and tends to regress in the postpartum period. Interestingly, researchers have found higher levels of prolactin and dopamine receptor (D2) in the myometrium of women with fibroids. This increased prolactin production in leiomyomas may stimulate transdifferentiation of myometrial cells to myofibroblasts contributing to the fibrogenicity of fibroids.[13] Moreover, myometrial cells with high levels of estrogens and progesterone receptors have been shown to stimulate the growth of adjuvant fibroid stem cells. In addition, somatic mutations (i.e., *MED 12*, *HMGA-1*, and *HMGA-2*) and some inherited mutations have been identified to be associated with fibroids.

TYPES OF FIBROIDS

Fibroids are traditionally classified as cervical, submucosal, subserosal, and intramural depending on their location. The International Federation of Gynaecology and Obstetrics (FIGO) PALM-COEIN (*p*olyp; *a*denomyosis; *l*eiomyoma; *m*alignancy and hyperplasia; *c*oagulopathy; *o*vulatory dysfunction; *e*ndometrial; *i*atrogenic; and *n*ot yet classified) classification systems[14] as shown in **Figure 1** have simplified the classification of fibroids and have been accepted internationally. The key point of FIGO staging is that it allows the allocation of a range of stages if the fibroid traverses multiple layers of the uterus; for instance, a fibroid extending from the cavity to the subserosal layer is labeled type 2–5. Such fibroids, namely hybrid fibroids, can contribute to subfertility.

Some ultrasound and MRI images of fibroids with their classification are given in **Figures 2 to 5**.

ARE ALL FIBROIDS ASSOCIATED WITH INFERTILITY?

All fibroids do not cause subfertility. Intracavitary fibroids indenting the cavity such as pedunculated submucous fibroids (FIGO 0), submucosal (SM) (FIGO 1) with <50% intramural and submucosal (FIGO 2) with >50% intramural can cause subfertility and can be removed by hysteroscopic myomectomy.[14,15] There is controversy regarding the removal of intramural fibroids just contacting the endometrium (FIGO 3), intramural (FIGO 4), and intramural with <50% subserosal (FIGO 5) fibroids.

Their removal depends on the size (>4 cm) and the clinical symptoms. Subserosal fibroids with <50% intramural (FIGO 6) and subserosal pedunculated (FIGO 7) can be left behind. Others such as cervical or parasitic fibroids (FIGO 8) usually do not impact fertility and hence can be left too.

Intramural fibroids away from the endometrial cavity or subserosal fibroids can be approached through the laparoscopic approach. A waiting period of at least 3 months is advised after myomectomy to

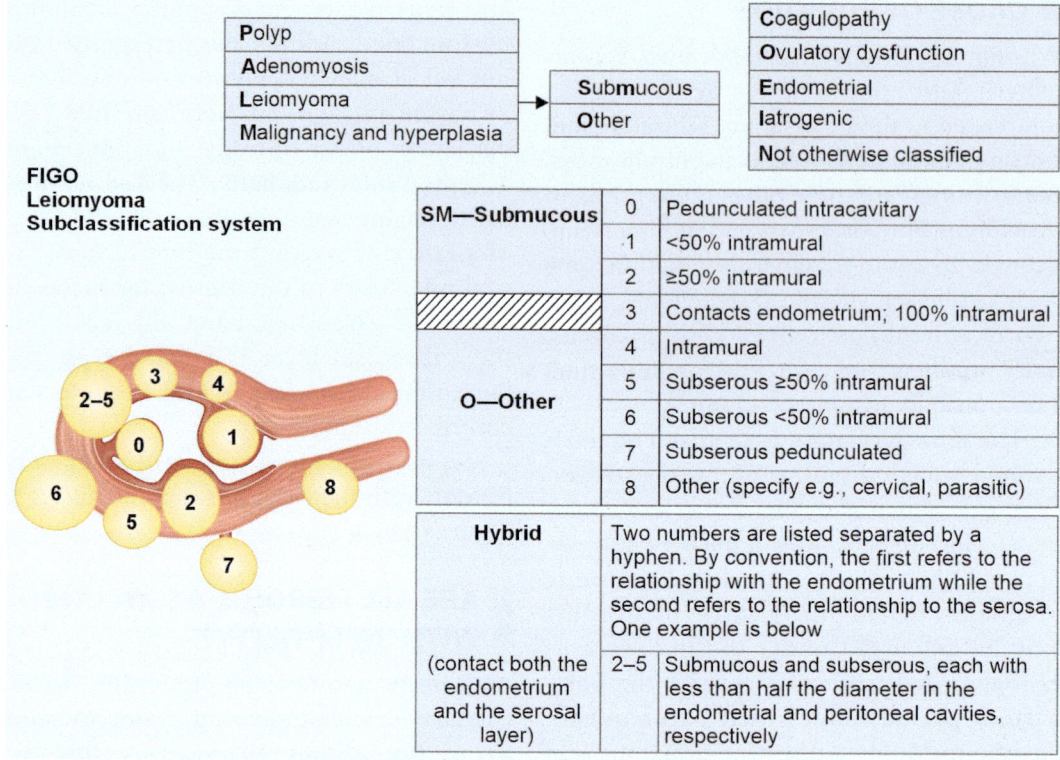

Fig. 1: FIGO PALM-COEIN classification system 2011. (FIGO: International Federation of Gynaecology and Obstetrics; PALM COEIN: *p*olyp; *a*denomyosis; *l*eiomyoma; *m*alignancy and hyperplasia; *c*oagulopathy; *o*vulatory dysfunction; *e*ndometrial; *i*atrogenic; and *n*ot yet classified)
Courtesy: Malcolm G Murray, MD.

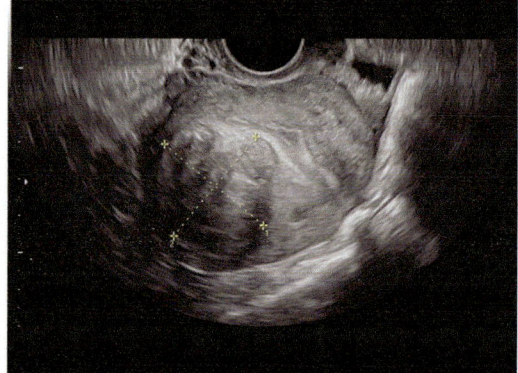

Fig. 2: USG image of intramural fibroid with submucosal component indenting the endometrial cavity measuring 3.69 × 3.59 cm (FIGO SM-2).

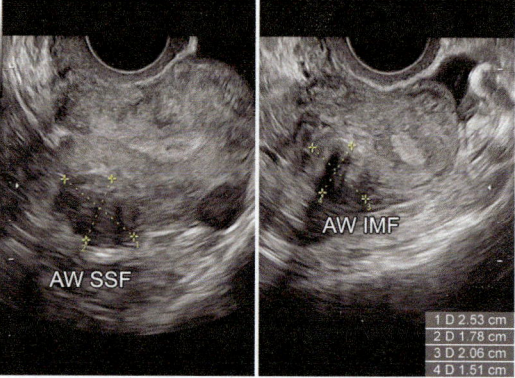

Fig. 3: USG image of posterior wall subserosal fibroid measuring 2.5 × 1.78 × 2.06 cm (FIGO 5).

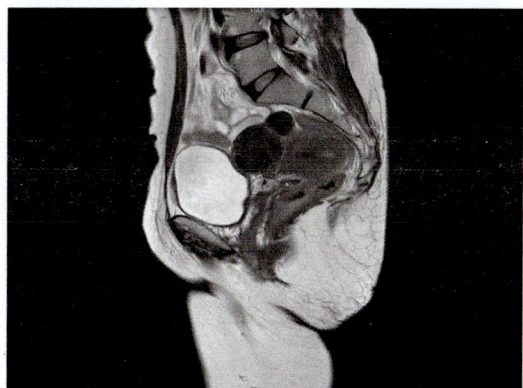

Fig. 4: MRI image of a fundal subserosal fibroid measuring 3.2 × 2.8 × 2.5 cm indenting the urinary bladder (FIGO 6). A second subserosal fibroid measuring 1.2 × 1.1 × 1.3 cm arising from the posterior wall is seen next to it (FIGO 6).

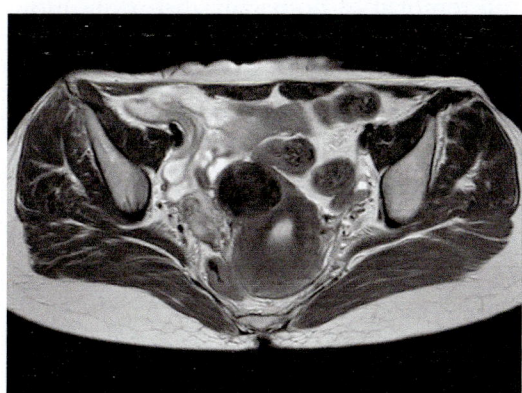

Fig. 5: MRI image of a subserosal anterior wall fibroid measuring 2.8 × 2.5 × 2.9 cm (FIGO type 6).

allow for the fibroid bed to heal before any infertility treatment.

A two-step approach is sometimes employed for hysteroscopic myomectomy for fibroids >3 cm or in the presence of multiple submucosal fibroids on opposing walls. A second approach is to give 2–3 months of gonadotrophin-releasing hormone or ulipristal acetate (UPA) to shrink the fibroid size before embarking on hysteroscopic myomectomy.

Abdominal myomectomy is reserved for patients with multiple fibroids, requiring multiple incisions, or for large fibroids (>7 cm) or suspected of being a leiomyosarcoma.

DOES THE SIZE OF THE FIBROID IMPACT FERTILITY?

Any fibroid >4 cm by its sheer size can affect the vascularity of the surrounding myometrium, affecting fertility, and hence warrants removal. This has been reiterated by various authors including Sunkara et al. in 2010.[16-18]

Somigliana et al.[4] in a meta-analysis proposed the removal of intracavitary fibroids and intramural fibroids >4 cm.[4]

IN VITRO FERTILIZATION OUTCOMES WITH FIBROIDS

Fibroids as space-occupying lesions (SOL) can affect the implantation of embryos in the uterus causing implantation failure and also the risk of subsequent miscarriage.

Pritts et al. analyzed 23 studies on in vitro fertilization (IVF)/intracytoplasmic sperm injection (ICSI) outcomes with fibroids and showed significantly reduced clinical pregnancy rates, implantation, ongoing pregnancy/live birth rates, and increased miscarriage rates with submucosal fibroids.[1]

Wang et al. in an updated meta-analysis on 9,189 IVF cycles also found significantly reduced clinical pregnancy rates, live birth rates, and increased miscarriage rates with fibroids.[19]

The Cochrane Review (2020) which included four randomized controlled trials (RCTs) and 442 participants found low-quality evidence in favor of myomectomy.[20] Furthermore, regarding the route of removal, the current evidence does not indicate a superior method (laparoscopy, laparotomy, or different electrosurgical systems) to improve rates of live birth rates, clinical pregnancy or ongoing pregnancy rates, or miscarriage rates.

ROLE OF MEDICAL MANAGEMENT OF FIBROIDS WITH INFERTILITY

The various medical options available for treating fibroids include the following:
- Magnetic resonance-guided focused ultrasound surgery (MRgFUS) is now finding its place in infertility associated with fibroids. This noninvasive option has a quick recovery time and a low risk of complications.[21]
- Radiofrequency ablation (RFA) is yet another alternative method wherein hyperthermic ablation is used to cause fibroid shrinkage. It can be combined with laparoscopic procedures and ultrasound guidance to shrink the fibroids.[22] Since the data comes from case reports and case series following the RFA trial for symptomatic fibroids, its use in infertility management awaits more studies.
- Uterine artery embolization (UAE) utilizes fluoroscopy to place embolic particles in the uterine circulation for occluding the blood flow to fibroids. However, this procedure carries a small risk of decreasing the blood flow to the ovaries and also carries a risk of causing pregnancy complications and hence is not recommended for infertile women.[23]

CONCLUSION

Leiomyoma are the most common benign tumors seen in women of reproductive age group (30–40%) with higher prevalence in infertile patients.

Fibroids impact fertility by interfering with sperm transport, ER, deranged cytokine profile, abnormal vascularization, chronic inflammation, increasing myometrial peristalsis, and thickening of the junctional zone, hence interfering with implantation rates and causing increased miscarriage rate.

What causes the fibroids to grow is largely unknown but there seem to be genetic and epigenetic factors responsible for it. Obesity, Black race, familial history, vitamin D deficiency, and a diet rich in animal fats are some of the risk factors.

The decision to operate on fibroids depends on their size, number, location, and their impact on fertility.

Surgical treatment still remains the mainstay of treatment for fibroids. Currently, hysteroscopic myomectomy is recommended for submucosal fibroids (FIGO 0, 1, 2, 3 fibroids). There is still controversy regarding the removal of noncavity-distorting intramural fibroids. Subserosal fibroids need not be removed as they do not impact fertility.

The size of the fibroid does matter. Intramural fibroids >4 cm should be removed. With the increasing use of ART, myomectomy prior to IVF is recommended for submucosal fibroids (FIGO 0 and 1).

Cochrane Review (2020) and the American Society of Reproductive Medicine (2017) recommend against the removal of noncavity-deforming myomas.

MRgFUS, a noninvasive method, as well as RFA's use in fibroids-associated infertility awaits further studies and cannot be recommended currently.

Considering the long-term effect of UAE on decreasing the blood supply to the uterus and ovaries, it is not recommended for infertility associated with fibroids.

REFERENCES

1. Pritts EA, Parker WH, Olive DL. Fibroids and infertility: an updated systematic review of the evidence. Fertil Steril. 2009;91:1215-23.
2. Fernandez H, Sefrioui, O, Virelizier C, Gervaise A, Gomel, V, Frydman, R. Hysteroscopic resection of submucosal myomas in

patients with infertility. Hum Reprod. 2001; 16:1489-92.
3. Goldenberg M, Sivan E, Sharabi Z, Bider D, Rabinovici J, Seidman DS. Outcome of hysteroscopic resection of submucous myomas for infertility. Fertil Steril. 1995; 64:714-6.
4. Somigliana E, Vercellini P, Daguati R, Pasin R, De Giorgi O, Crosignani PG. Fibroids and female reproduction: a critical analysis of the evidence. Hum Reprod. 2007;13:465-76.
5. Pier BD, Bates GW. Potential causes of subfertility in patients with intramural fibroids. Fertil Res Pract. 2015;1:12.
6. Lash GE, Bulmer JN. Do uterine natural killer (uNK) cells contribute to female reproductive disorders? J Reprod Immunol. 2011:88:156-64.
7. Ciavattini A, Giuseppe JD, Stortoni P, Montik N, Giannubilo SR, Litta P, et al. Uterine fibroids: Pathogenesis and interactions with endometrium and endomyometrial junction. Obstet Gynecol Int 2013;2013:173184.
8. Yoshino O, Hayashi T, Osuga Y, Orisaka M, Asada H, Okuda S, et al. Decreased pregnancy rate is linked to abnormal uterine peristalsis caused by intramural fibroids. Hum Reprod. 2010;25:2475-9.
9. Tinelli A, Mynbaev OA, Mettler L, Hurst BS, Pellegrino M, Nicolardi G, et al. A combined ultrasound and histologic approach for analysis of uterine fibroid pseudocapsule thickness. Reprod Sci. 2014:21:1177-86.
10. Baranov VS, Osinovskaya NS, Yarmolinskaya MI. Pathogenomics of uterine fibroids development. Int J Mol Sci. 2019; 20(24):6151.
11. Islam MS, Akhtar MM, Segars JH. Vitamin D deficiency and uterine fibroids: an opportunity for treatment or prevention? Fertil Steril. 2021;115:1175-6.
12. Vergara D, Catherino WH, Trojano G, Tinelli A. Vitamin D: mechanism of action and biological effects in uterine fibroids. Nutrients. 2021;13:597.
13. DiMauro A, Seger C, Minor B, Amitrano AM, Okeke I, Taya M, et al. Prolactin is expressed in uterine leiomyomas and promotes signaling and fibrosis in myometrial cells. Reprod Sci. 2021;29(9):2525-35.
14. Munro MG, Critchley HO, Broder MS, Fraser IS; FIGO Working Group on Menstrual Disorders. FIGO classification system (PALM-COEIN) for causes of abnormal uterine bleeding in nongravid women of reproductive age. Int J Gynaecol Obstet. 2011;113(1):3-13.
15. Casadio P, Guasina F, Morra C, Talamo MT, Leggieri C, Frisoni J, et al. Hysteroscopic myomectomy: techniques and preoperative assessment. Minerva Ginecol. 2016;68: 154-66.
16. Sunkara SK, Khairy M, El-Toukhy T, Khalaf Y, Coomarasamy A. The effect of intramural fibroids without uterine cavity involvement on the outcome of IVF treatment: a systematic review and meta-analysis. Hum Reprod. 2010;25(2):418-29.
17. Casini ML, Casini ML, Rossi F, Agostini R, Unfer V. Effects of the position of fibroids on fertility. Gynecol Endocrinol. 2006;22(2):106-9.
18. Oliveira FG, Abdelmassih VG, Diamond MP, Dozortsev D, Melo NR, Abdelmassih R. Impact of subserosal and intramural uterine fibroids that do not distort the endometrial cavity on the outcome of in vitro fertilization-intracytoplasmic sperm injection. Fertil Steril. 2004;81(3):582-7.
19. Wang X, Chen L, Wang H, Li Q, Liu X, Qi H. The impact of noncavity-distorting intramural fibroids on the efficacy of in vitro fertilization-embryo transfer: an updated meta-analysis. BioMed Res Int. 2018; 8924703:1-13.
20. Metwally M, Raybould G, Cheong YC, Horne AW. Surgical treatment of fibroids for subfertility. Cochrane Database Syst Rev. 2020;1(1):CD003857.
21. Jeng CJ, Ou KY, Long CY, Chuang L, Ker CR, 500 Cases of high-intensity focused ultrasound (HIFU) ablated uterine fibroids and adenomyosis. Taiwan J Obs Gynecol. 2020;59:865-71.
22. Lee BB, Yu SP. Radiofrequency ablation of uterine fibroids: a review. Curr Obstet Gynecol Rep. 2016;5:318-24.
23. Karlsen K, Hrobjartsson A, Korsholm M, Mogensen O, Humaidan P, Ravn P. Fertility after uterine artery embolization of fibroids: a systematic review. Arch Gynecol Obstet. 2018:297:13-25.

CHAPTER 5

Fibroids and Abnormal Uterine Bleeding Patterns

Shehla Jamal

■ INTRODUCTION

Abnormal uterine bleeding (AUB) is a profound gynecological entity, and the major manifestation is heavy menstrual blood (HMB) loss affecting 14–25% of women of reproductive age and poses a countable impact on their physical, social, emotional, and day-to-day quality of life.[1]

Fibroids or leiomyomas are the most commonly detected tumors of the uterus. It is reported to contribute to abnormal bleeding in nearly 70% white females and >80% of African females will receive a diagnosis of fibroid by the end of perimenopause.[2]

In India, approximately 30% of the females in the reproductive age group have AUB is associated with fibroids. Around 33% of gynecological surgeries are attributed to symptomatic fibroids.[3]

■ SYMPTOMATOLOGY OF FIBROIDS

Around 46–50% of the fibroids are asymptomatic and are an incidental finding on imaging for other conditions. Symptomatic leiomyomas are often seen with subfertility, miscarriage, preterm labor, and obstructed labor. Additionally, they may cause dragging sensation and pelvic pressure symptoms **(Table 1)**.

Abnormal uterine bleeding was rechristened by Fédération International de Gynécologie et d'Obstétrique (FIGO) by the FIGO Menstrual Disorders Group in 2009 and Leiomyoma subclassification was also introduced **(Fig. 1)**.[4]

This subclassification helped in understanding the menstrual pattern disturbance and designing the management approach more accurately.

■ MOLECULAR AND BIOCHEMICAL CAUSES OF ABNORMAL UTERINE BLEEDING WITH FIBROIDS

Although the association between AUB and fibroids remains incompletely worked up many plausible explanations have been submitted from time to time. The observed paradox is that some women having fibroids have entirely normal bleeding patterns.

Previously presented theories explain an increased endometrial surface area and the presence of fragile and engorged blood vessels in the endomyometrial junction. The exaggerated turbulent vascular flow observed in these enlarged vessels alters platelet action, thus causing heavy bleeding.[5] The newer perspectives regarding the cellular and molecular alterations associated with fibroids can have an impact on angiogenesis,

TABLE 1: Varied symptomatology of fibroids.		
Location of fibroid	*Symptom*	*Common presentation*
• Subserosal (FIGO types 6, 7) • Placed anteriorly	• Usually asymptomatic • Pelvic pressure • Frequency of micturition • Recurrent UTI	Pelvic mass
• Subserosal (FIGO types 6, 7) • Placed posteriorly	• Low backache • Constipation • Rectal tenesmus • Deep dyspareunia	Irregular uterine enlargement
• Subserosal and Intramural (FIGO types 4, 5, 6, 7) • Placed laterally	• Recurrent UTI • Hydronephrosis • Pyonephrosis • Thromboembolism	Adenomyomas as important differential
Intramural (FIGO types 4, 5)	• Usually asymptomatic • Pressure symptoms	Irregular to diffuse uterine enlargement
Intramural and subserosal (FIGO types 0, 1, 2, 2–5)	Symptoms-related uterine bleeding	Bulky uterus, HMB, and associated anemia

(FIGO: Fédération International de Gynécologie et d'Obstétrique; HMB: heavy menstrual bleeding; UTI: urinary tract infection)

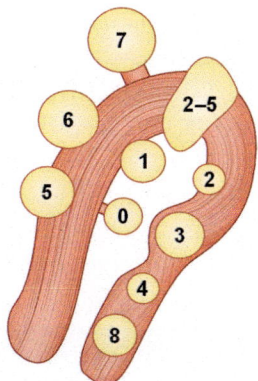

Fig. 1: FIGO subclassification for leiomyoma.

alteration in vasoactive substances, and growth factors as well as disturb the coagulation mechanisms.[6]

Some authors have suggested an increased level of matrix metalloproteinase (MMP) 2 and 11, but the precise impact on increased endometrial bleeding is still unclear. Other vascular-expressed factors, such as vascular endothelial growth factor (VEGF), basic fibroblast growth factor (bFGF), platelet-derived growth factor (PDGF), and parathyroid hormone-related protein (PTHrP), all have potential angiogenic effects but their specific role in HMB is still unexplored.[7]

TOPOGRAPHIC ASSOCIATION OF ABNORMAL UTERINE BLEEDING WITH FIBROIDS

Submucosal

The location of fibroids, especially submucosal (SM) fibroids deforming the cavity is more likely to present with HMB flow. There is a current bifurcation of opinion that women with significant cavity distortion represent additional diagnostic and therapeutic challenges.

Submucosal and intramural fibroids can induce mechanotransductional changes which result in myometrial rigidity and reduced myometrial contractility, affecting endometrial bleeding[8] **(Fig. 2)**.

Observed patterns in the case of SM fibroids are as follows:
- HMB due to increased surface area, perilesional endometrial hyperplasia, hypervascularization
- Intermenstrual bleeding (IMB) due to venous congestion and surface fragility
- Prolonged menstrual bleeding due to venous microulceration
- Heavy and prolonged bleeding.

They have a serially increasing blood loss graph and have the notoriety of responding very poorly to medical management. The dreaded challenge is faced in managing adolescent SM fibroids.

The STEP-W classification and management algorithm are quite widely accepted for formulating a management approach in the SM variety of leiomyomas[9] **(Table 2)**.

Fibroid Polyp

Fibroid polyps are a type 0 class of leiomyomas, a name ascribed to the presence of a connecting stalk between the fibroid mass and endomyometrium. There is dependent vascular congestion in these fibroid polyps and the surface is usually very congested and fragile. They tend to get inflamed and infected very easily **(Figs. 3A and B)**.

The common AUB pattern loss observed is:
- HMB attributed to the highly vascular and large surface
- Acyclic IMB because of venous and capillary fragility
- Postcoital bleeding (if protruding out of external os) as there is trauma and infection
- Prolonged menstrual bleeding

The diagnostic suspicion is raised when the *classic presentation* of acyclic

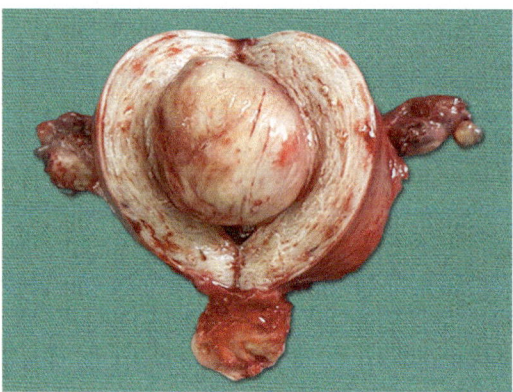

Fig. 2: Submucosal fibroid.

TABLE 2: STEP-W classification and management of fibroids.

	Size (cm)	Topography	Extension of the base	Penetration	Lateral wall	Total
0	<2	Low	<1/3	0	+1	
1	2–5	Middle	1/3–2/3	<50%		
2	>5	Upper	>2/3	>50%		
Score		**Group**	**Complexity and management approach**			
0–4		1	Low-complexity hysteroscopic myomectomy			
5–6		2	High-complexity hysteroscopic myomectomy, GnRH, two-step myomectomy			
7–9		3	Consider alternatives to hysteroscopic approach			

(GnRH: gonadotropin-releasing hormone; STEP-W: severity, timing, endometrial evaluation, polyp and fibroid assessment-work up for coagulation disorders)

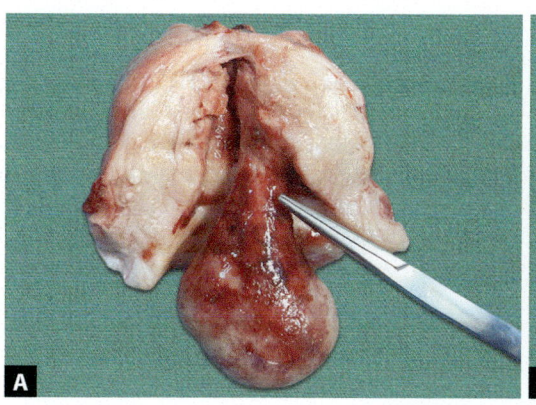
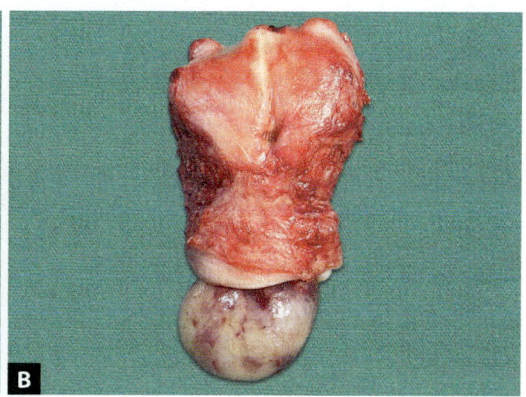

Figs. 3A and B: Fibroid polyp.

IMB is evaluated. As presumed, they also do not respond to medical management and warrant a polypectomy for symptom resolution. Hysteroscopic aid is much beneficial to locate the pedicle, to minimize the recurrence risk. Some clinicians prefer gonadotropin-releasing hormone (GnRH) analog pretreatment to reduce blood loss.[10]

Intramural

Such fibroids can also cause a variety of symptoms related to bleeding. Surface area expansion, altered myometrial contractility around fibroids, associated endometrial hyperplasia, and altered coagulation mechanism can lead to episodes of heavy bleeding.[11]

The usual patterns are:
- Heavy, cyclical bleeding as they are largely contained in the mural segment of the uterus
- Heavy prolonged cyclical bleeding due to increased vascularity
- HMB associated with dysmenorrhea as the entrapped fibroids have shown an increased amount of prostaglandins compared to normal endometrium.

They respond quite well to medical management as well as levonorgestrel intrauterine system (LNG-IUS) when the cavity contour is maintained.

■ CONCLUSION

Identification of AUB pattern gives a good clue to make the diagnosis of the fibroids which in turn serves to tailor the best investigation and treatment strategy for the patients. Exploring new mechanisms associated with AUB (L) will open up the range of therapeutic options for the clinicians as sometimes age and parity profile limits therapeutic options.

■ REFERENCES

1. Vaidya R, Vinayachandran S, Devi S, Prejisha B, Lekshminath G, Sreedharan S, et al. Prevalence of abnormal uterine bleeding and its associated risk factors in women of perimenopausal age group – A retrospective Study 59994_CE(Vi). J Clin Diagn Res. 2022; 16(12):QC09-13.
2. Whitaker L, Critchley HOD. Abnormal uterine bleeding. Best Pract Res Clin Obstet Gynaecol. 2016;34:54-65.
3. Sharma A, Dogra Y. Trends of AUB in tertiary centre of Shimla hills. J Midlife Health. 2013;4(1):67-8.
4. Munro MG, Critchley HOD, Fraser IS; FIGO Menstrual Disorders Committee. The two FIGO systems for normal and abnormal uterine bleeding symptoms and classification

of causes of abnormal uterine bleeding in the reproductive years: 2018 revisions. Int J Gynaecol Obstet. 2018;143(3):393-408. [Erratum in: Int J Gynaecol Obstet. 2019; 144(2):237.]
5. Stewart EA, Nowak RA. Leiomyoma-related bleeding: a classic hypothesis updated for the molecular era. Hum Reprod Update. 1996;2:295-306.
6. Munro MG. Classification of menstrual bleeding disorders. Rev Endocr Metab Disord. 2012;13:225-34.
7. Palmer SS, Haynes-Johnson D, Diehl T, Nowak RA. Increased expression of stromelysin 3 mRNA in leiomyomas (uterine fibroids) compared with myometrium. J Soc Gynecol Investig. 1998;5:203-9.
8. Szamatowicz J, Laudanski T, Bulkszas B, Akerlund M. Fibromyomas and uterine contractions. Acta Obstet Gynecol Scand. 1997;76(10):973-6.
9. Lasmar RB, Lasmar BP, Celeste RK, da Rosa DB, Depes de B, Lopes RG. A new system to classify submucous myomas: a Brazilian multicenter study. J Minim Invasive Gynecol. 2012;19(5):575-80.
10. Sun P, Dong Y, Yu Y, Xu H, Zhu L, Zhang P, et al. Gonadotropin-releasing hormone agonist (GnRH-a) pretreatment before hormone replacement therapy does not improve reproductive outcomes of frozen-thawed embryo transfer cycle in older patients with intrauterine fibroid: a retrospective cohort study. J Clin Med. 2023;12(4):1401.
11. Henderson D. The incidence of endometrial hyperplasia with uterine fibroids and external and internal endometriosis (adenomyosis). Am J Obstet Gynecol. 1941;41(4):694-7.

CHAPTER 6

Secondary Changes in Fibroid

Prerna Keshan

■ INTRODUCTION

Being the most common benign tumor of the reproductive age-group, fibroids generally lack malignant potential. However, secondary changes might occur in these benign lesions that may cause diagnostic issues because of other mimicking conditions on routine ultrasonography. Such changes must be kept in mind and treatment modality standardized accordingly to avoid unnecessary surgical interventions. Treatment of fibroids with secondary changes depends on the age, reproductive desires, symptoms, and relevant associated physiological conditions.

■ BACKGROUND

Throughout the yesteryears, it has been well known that the secondary changes in fibroids may aggravate symptoms of pain and discomfort in females. Hence, every woman detected with a fibroid should be counseled in complete detail about the possible secondary changes in due course of time if conservative management for fibroids is opted for. To avoid undue apprehension in case an acute secondary change occurs, proper information about the same on the day of diagnosis of a fibroid may pave the way toward a better understanding of the treatment modality by the patient.

Types of Secondary Changes

Types of secondary changes are:
- Hemorrhage
- Hydropic
- Myxoid
- Necrosis
- Calcification
- Atrophy
- Infection
- Vascular changes
- *Sarcomatous changes:* Incidence of sarcomatous transformation in benign uterine leiomyomas is reported to be 0.1–0.8%
- Degenerative changes.

Degenerative Changes

Degenerative changes are considered to arise from exponential growth that outmatches the blood supply or mechanical compression of the feeder arteries.
- *Hyaline degeneration:* It is a common degeneration occurring in around 57.9% of fibroids wherein the firm feel of the tumor becomes soft and elastic due to the accumulation of extracellular matrix.
- *Cystic degeneration:* It occurs in around 7.2% of patients usually after menopause, in cases of interstitial fibroids. Liquefication of areas with hyaline changes may be confused with ovarian cysts or pregnancy.

- Fatty degeneration occurs at or after menopause wherein fat globules get deposited in the muscle cells.
- *Subserosal fibroid (sequence of events):* Pedunculated-torsion-acute abdominal pain-detachment-wandering fibroid-attachment to another peritoneal structure-parasite fibroid.
- Saponification
- *Red degeneration (aseptic necrobiosis):*[1] It is also known as carneous degeneration. It occurs in around 8% of tumors complicating pregnancy and prevalent in 3% of all uterine leiomyomas. It usually occurs in large fibroids. While it is an uncommon type of degenerative, it is considered the most common during pregnancy.

Pathology of red degeneration:[2] This is a subtype of hemorrhagic infarction that often occurs in the pregnant state. On gross pathology, it is characterized by the red (hemorrhagic) appearance of the leiomyoma. Red degeneration primarily occurs secondary to venous thrombosis within the periphery of the tumor or rupture of intratumoral arteries.

Microscopic examination reveals numerous dilated thrombosed vessels filled with red cells at the periphery. These red blood cells in the thrombosed vessels have abundant levels of intracellular methemoglobin.

- *MRI findings:*[3] Hyperintense signal on T1W1 and hypointense signal on T2W1
- *Laboratory investigations:* Usually reveal an increase in white blood cell count and anemia in cases of vaginal bleeding.

Symptoms of red degeneration:
- *Severe pain:* Pain is the most frequent sign of uterine leiomyoma degeneration. It is often severe and localized to the site of the fibroid. Severe pain usually lasts for 2–4 weeks.
- Vomiting
- Vaginal bleeding
- Nausea
- Fever is usually low grade.

Treatment of red degeneration:[4]
- Rest
- Adequate hydration
- Hospitalization due to fear of preterm labor
- Sedation
- Anti-inflammatory.

Observant attitude is usually undertaken apart from a few more intractable cases where surgical intervention is required.

CONCLUSION

Although leiomyomas are the most common benign solid tumors of the reproductive age group, not much research has been done in this aspect of secondary changes in the lesions. Larger cohort studies are required to come to a specific conclusion on the risk factors and predisposing causes of such secondary metamorphosis. The presence of secondary changes poses a significant problem in the establishment of differential diagnosis with malignant transformation even in advanced diagnostic modalities like MRI. Hence, utmost caution should be taken while considering a secondary change in fibroid and vouching the diagnosis accordingly. Since an expectant attitude is usually undertaken for asymptomatic fibroids, degenerative changes may compel the care provider to take aggressive surgical interventions if proper counseling is lacking.

REFERENCES

1. Kawakami S, Togashi K, Konishi I, Kimura I, Fukuoka M, Mori T, et al. Red degeneration of uterine leiomyoma: MR appearance. J Comput Assist Tomogr. 1994;18(6):925-8.

2. Murase E, Siegelman ES, Outwater EK, Perez-Jaffe LA, Tureck RW. Uterine leiomyomas: histopathologic features, MR imaging findings, differential diagnosis, and treatment. Radiographics. 1999;19(5):1179-97.
3. Okizuka H, Sugimura K, Takemori M, Obayashi C, Kitao M, Ishida T. MR detection of degenerating uterine leiomyomas. J Comput Assist Tomogr. 1993;17(5):760-6.
4. Ueda H, Togashi K, Konishi I, Kataoka ML, Koyama T, Fujiwara T, et al. Unusual appearances of uterine leiomyomas: MR imaging findings and their histopathologic backgrounds. Radiographics. 1999;19 Spec No:S131-45.

CHAPTER 7

Medical Management of Fibroids

Upma Saxena, Monika Rana

■ INTRODUCTION

Fibroids are benign, monoclonal tumors of the smooth muscle cells of the myometrium containing large aggregations of extracellular matrix composed of collagen, elastin, fibronectin and proteoglycan. The exact cause of uterine fibroids is unknown, but they have been associated with increased estrogen levels. They are more commonly observed in individuals of reproductive age, and approximately one in three women will develop uterine fibroids during their lifetime. The incidence of fibroids tends to increase with age until menopause, with a peak occurrence in their 40s, after which they typically decrease in size.[1]

Treatment options for heavy menstrual bleeding (HMB) due to fibroids should take into account their size, number, and location, a woman's fertility preferences, any comorbidities, the presence or absence of polyps, endometrial pathology or adenomyosis, and presence of symptoms such as pressure and pain. When no associated cause is identified and fibroids are <3 cm in diameter, pharmacotherapy is recommended for symptomatic relief. This may include nonhormonal treatments such as tranexamic acid and nonsteroidal anti-inflammatory drugs (NSAIDs), as well as hormonal treatments such as combined hormonal contraception (CHC), cyclical oral progestogens, and levonorgestrel intrauterine system (LNG-IUS).

Nonsurgical options such as uterine artery embolization (UAE)[2] and magnetic resonance-guided focused ultrasound (MRgFUS) are preferred over ulipristal which is a selective progesterone receptor modulator (SPRM) because of the risk of severe hepatic toxicity. Hence, selecting the most conservative options that minimize morbidity and risk while optimizing outcomes is crucial, especially when managing this condition. This principal approach ensures that patients receive effective treatment with the least possible impact on their health and well-being. By carefully weighing the benefits and risks of different treatment options, healthcare providers can tailor management strategies to meet the individual needs of each patient.[3]

Indeed, controlling menstrual blood loss is often considered the most clinically important aspect of managing uterine fibroids. By effectively reducing menstrual bleeding loss (MBL), the risk of anemia can be minimized, and the overall quality of life (QoL) for individuals affected by fibroids can be significantly improved. Ensuring optimal menstrual management is essential for enhancing patient well-being and addressing the associated physical and emotional impacts of HMB.[4]

Surgical options, i.e., endometrial ablation and hysterectomy, should be offered only when pharmacological and nonsurgical alternative treatments have failed or been refused by patient or patient has serious symptoms. Medical management in some cases can reduce the need for surgery, but often it is not a lifelong solution and is effective mainly for myoma <3 cm. Myoma >3 cm needs fertility-preserving myomectomy, which can be done by abdominal, vaginal, hysteroscopic, and laparoscopic routes. Various treatment options are shown in **Figure 1**.

Donnez and coworkers conducted an analysis comparing the benefits of both medical and surgical therapies for the management of fibroids and have proposed new comprehensive guidelines for fibroid management, taking into account specific symptoms such as bleeding, infertility, and the patient's age.[5] The efficacy of pharmacological treatments for HMB may be limited in women with fibroids that are substantially >3 cm in diameter.[4]

Indications of medical therapy are:
- To improve menorrhagia
- To correct anemia before surgery
- Presurgical to decrease size and vascularity of tumor in order to facilitate surgery so that hysterectomy can be done vaginally, i.e., nondecent vaginal hysterectomy (NDVH), or Pfannenstiel incision can be used instead of vertical incision while performing abdominal hysterectomy.
- Alternative to surgery in perimenopausal woman with high risk factors for surgery
- Temporary postponement of surgery

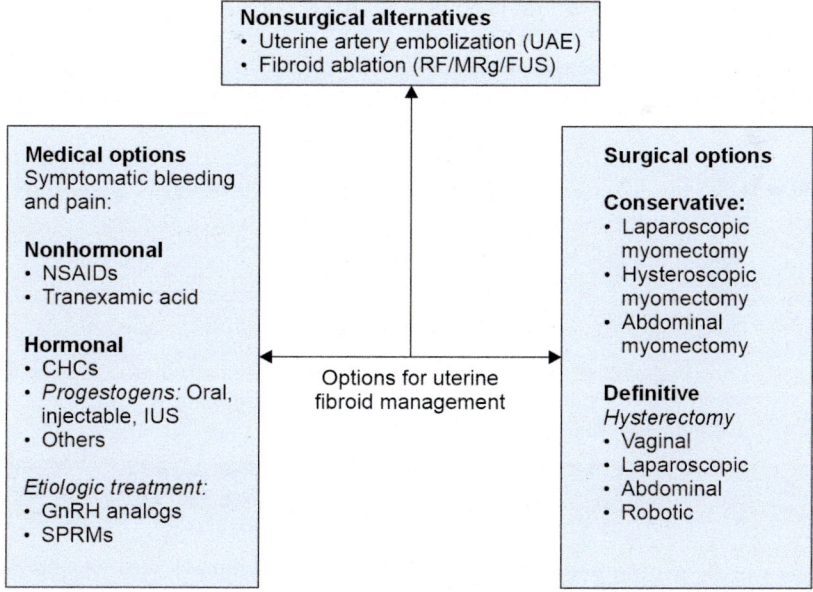

Fig. 1: Surgical, nonsurgical, and medical therapy currently used for the management of uterine fibroids. (CHCs: combined hormonal contraceptives; GnRH: gonadotropin-releasing hormone; IUS: intrauterine system; MRgFUS: magnetic resonance-guided focused ultrasound surgery; NSAIDs: nonsteroidal anti-inflammatory drugs; RF: radiofrequency ablation; SPRMs: selective progesterone receptor modulators; UAE: uterine artery embolization)

In a systematic review, 75 randomized controlled trials (RCTs) were evaluated, leading to the conclusion that there was insufficient evidence to recommend any particular medical treatment for fibroid. However, it was noted that the overall quality of the studies reviewed was very low.[6]

Conversely, another systematic review conducted in the same year analyzed 52 studies and concluded that there was sufficient evidence supporting the efficacy of medical alternatives to surgery for fibroids.[7]

NONHORMONAL TREATMENT (TABLE 1)

Nonsteroidal Anti-inflammatory Drugs

Nonsteroidal anti-inflammatory drugs work by decreasing the production of prostaglandins and causing uterine vasoconstriction. Their efficacy in reducing MBL varies widely depending on factors such as the type of NSAID, dosage used, and duration of use. Clinical studies have reported MBL reduction ranging from 10 to 55% with their use.[4,8,9]

Indications for NSAID are as follows:
- As an interim measure while awaiting investigations or alternative treatments are being contemplated
- When fertility preservation is necessary
- Where hormonal treatments are leading to side effects
- When pain is the patient's biggest concern

Nonsteroidal anti-inflammatory drugs are typically used only during menstruation and are most effective in patients with a regular monthly cycle. They can reduce both bleeding and pain and are nonhormonal, thus not affecting fertility. They are taken orally, starting from day 1 of the menstrual cycle or just before periods, until HMB has ceased. Studies have shown similar efficacy for NSAIDs such as mefenamic acid, diclofenac,

TABLE 1: Summary of medical therapy.

Types of drug	Drugs	Outcome of fibroid size	Outcome on abnormal uterine bleeding	Outcome on fertility
Nonhormonal	NSAIDs and tranexamic acid	No effect on fibroid size	Decrease by 30%	No effect
Hormonal	CHC	No data	Decrease 20–30%	Contraceptive
	Oral progestins	Decrease 30%	Decrease >60%	Contraceptive
	LARC [e.g., Depo-medroxyprogesterone acetate (Provera)]	Decrease uterine volume by 35%	Break through bleeding	Contraceptive
	LNG-IUS (e.g., Mirena)	Decrease 20–30%	Decrease 40% Systemic side effects	Contraceptive
	GnRHa (3–6 months' duration of therapy)	• Decrease 30% • Decrease uterine volume by 35%	Decrease >80%	Contraceptive

(CHC: combined hormonal contraceptive; GnRHa: gonadotropin-releasing hormone agonist; LARC: long-acting reversible contraceptive; LNG-IUS: levonorgestrel intrauterine system; NSAIDs: nonsteroidal anti-inflammatory drugs)

and naproxen, with MBL reduction ranging from 24.6% to 30.2%.[8]

Mefenamic acid is the most commonly used NSAID, in the dose of 150–600 mg for 3–5 days. It can cause indigestion, diarrhea, and cardiovascular problems. There are chances of decline in its efficacy and being ineffective in HMB. There is a decrease in bleeding by 30% with no reduction in the size of the fibroid.

Tranexamic Acid (Antifibrinolytic)

Tranexamic acid functions as a competitive inhibitor of plasminogen activation, thereby acting as an antifibrinolytic agent. Its efficacy in reducing MBL depends on the treatment regimen and duration of use. It has been found to have a slightly better effect on reduction of MBL compared to NSAIDs, although it does not impact pain associated with menstruation.

The recommended dosage of tranexamic acid is 1 g orally three times daily, starting on day 1 of the menstrual cycle and continuing for up to 4–5 days. With long-term use (over 2 years), it has been shown to achieve sustained improvements in the QoL for patients experiencing HMB.[8] Its common side effects are stomach upset, diarrhea, and headaches. It can lead to serious ocular changes in color vision/visual acuity.

Indications of tranexamic acid are as follows:[4,8,9]
- As a temporary measure while further investigations or alternative treatments are being organized
- When fertility is desired
- In cases where hormonal treatments causing side effects or are contraindicated
- When there are no structural uterine abnormalities or fibroids <3 cm

Tranexamic acid has rapid onset of action, no contraceptive effect, and no effect on the size of myoma. It is important to note that treatment with NSAIDs or tranexamic acid should be discontinued if no symptomatic improvement is observed within three menstrual cycles. While it can effectively reduce MBL, it does not address pain associated with menstruation. Additionally, it is contraindicated in patients with a history of thrombosis due to its anticoagulant properties.[3,4,8] Close monitoring of symptoms and patient response is essential to determine the effectiveness of treatment and to ensure patient safety. If symptoms persist or worsen, alternative treatment options should be considered in consultation with a healthcare provider.

HORMONAL TREATMENT (TABLE 1)

Combined Hormonal Contraceptives

Combined hormonal contraceptives is combination of estrogen and progesterone and oral dosing regimen include 21/7 and 24/4 for 6 months cyclically.[4] Suppress ovulation and prevent endometrial proliferation, inducing endometrial atrophy and decreasing prostaglandin production. The use of CHCs has been shown to lead to reductions in MBL of up to 43% at 3 months. Estradiol valerate/dienogest (E2V/DNG), when used for the treatment of HMB, can reduce median MBL by 88%.

However, it is important to note that the use of CHCs should be guided by the World Health Organization (WHO) medical eligibility criteria (MEC) for contraceptive use. While CHCs have a contraceptive effect, they do not impact future fertility.[4,9]

Common side effects of CHCs include mood changes, headaches, nausea, fluid retention, and breast tenderness. Patients should be aware of these potential side effects when considering CHCs for the management of HMB.[4,9]

Progestogens

High-dose Oral Progestogens

Only high-dose progestogens can be used in isolation, i.e., norethisterone acetate 5 mg or medroxyprogesterone acetate (MPA) 10 mg twice daily for ≥3 weeks (D5–D25) for 6 months.[8]

Long-course oral progestogens act by suppressing ovulation and preventing endometrial proliferation. Studies have shown that these medications can lead to reductions in MBL ranging from 32% to 78%. Typically, bleeding is regulated after—one to two cycles of treatment. Additionally, they can help achieve menstrual regularity in women with anovulatory bleeding.

When taken orally, long-course oral progestogens reduce bleeding but do not have an effect on fibroid size. Therefore, while they are effective in managing HMB, they do not directly address the underlying fibroids themselves. These medications are commonly used as a conservative treatment option for patients seeking symptom relief without surgical intervention.

Patients considering the use of long-course oral progestogens should be counseled about the possibility of experiencing amenorrhea, as up to 50% of women discontinue use within 1 year, with altered bleeding patterns being the most common reason for discontinuation. Compared to the LNG-IUS, long-course oral progestogens have lower patient satisfaction rates and lack long-term (>12 months) data on efficacy and safety.

Common side effects of long-course oral progestogens include weight gain, irregular bleeding, amenorrhea, and premenstrual-like syndrome symptoms such as bloating, fluid retention, and breast tenderness. Less common side effects include a small loss of bone mineral density (BMD), although this is typically reversible upon discontinuation of treatment. Patients should be informed about these potential side effects when considering a long course of oral progestogens for the management of HMB.[4,8]

Injectable Progestogens

Medroxyprogesterone acetate (Depo-Provera) which is also a long-acting reversible contraceptive (LARC) is administered as 150 mg intramuscular injection given 3 monthly and is devoid of any estrogenic side effects.[8,10] Progestogen-only implants are not advocated for the treatment of HMB. High-dose progesterone suppresses ovulation and prevents endometrial proliferation. Depo-Provera hinders fertility, which may take up to 12 months to return.[4,8]

LNG-IUS (Mirena/Medicated IUS)

The LNG-IUS is suitable for the treatment of HMB caused by fibroids when the uterine size is less than that of a 12-week pregnancy, and there is no distortion of the uterine cavity by the fibroids. This device slowly releases 20 µg of levonorgestrel directly into the endometrium every day, which prevents endometrial proliferation and reduces mean uterine vascular density.

Studies have shown that the LNG-IUS can reduce MBL by up to 96%, with a range of 71–96%, and this effect can last for up to 5 years. However, it is important to note that while the IUS effectively reduces bleeding, it has not been proven effective in reducing the size of the fibroids. Therefore, it is primarily used for managing HMB associated with fibroids rather than directly treating the fibroids.[8]

Levonorgestrel-releasing IUS is recommended as the first-line treatment for HMB in women with:[4]
- No identified pathology
- Fibroids <3 cm in diameter, which are not causing distortion of the uterine cavity
- Suspected or diagnosed adenomyosis

It reduces the need for surgery or other medical treatment but has contraceptive effect. Levonorgestrel-releasing intrauterine system (Mirena) is licensed only for treating HMB but not for the management of fibroid. Its use significantly elevates the levels of hemoglobin and ferritin. It is comparable to hysterectomy or endometrial ablation in causing significant improvement in QoL for 5-7 years without impairing future fertility.[8,11-13]

Levonorgestrel-releasing IUS leads to amenorrhea at 6 and 12 months in 65% and 48% women, respectively. The risk of uterine perforation and expulsion is 0.14% and 1.0%, respectively. EURAS-IUD reported a much higher expulsion rate in the HMB patients versus general population.[8,11-13]

The disadvantages of LNG-IUS when used in patients with fibroid are as follows:
- Does not significantly reduce fibroid volume
- Higher expulsion rates and irregular bleeding
- Cannot be used in large myomas distorting cavity

The side effects of LNG-IUS include irregular bleeding, i.e., spotting, oligomenorrhea, and amenorrhea, which can last up to 6 months. It also causes hormone-related problems such as acne, headache, and breast tenderness which, if present, are generally minor and transient but in rare cases period may stop altogether.

GONADOTROPIN-RELEASING HORMONE AGONIST (TABLE 2)

Gonadotropin-releasing hormone agonist (GnRHa) is a synthetic drug similar to hypothalamic GnRH in humans. It is given as a monthly injection for 3-6 months.[8] It suppresses estrogen and progesterone production and stops bleeding completely in 89% of women. It causes fibroid shrinkage by targeting the growth effects of estrogens and progesterone. GnRHa also relieves dysmenorrhea due to adenomyosis and endometriosis. The Food and Drug Administration (FDA) has approved the following GnRHa for preoperative use:
- *Inj. Leuprolide acetate:* 3.75 mg/month or 11.25 mg 3 monthly IM
- *Inj. Goserelin:* 3.6 mg/month or 10.8 mg 3 monthly SC depot implant
- *Inj. Triptorelin:* 3.75 mg/month or 11.25 mg 3 monthly IM

They are given for 6 months and the effect is seen in 3 months. There is an initial flare for 1 week followed by downregulation of the gonadotropin receptors in the pituitary. The initial flare phenomenon immediately following injection, which can cause worsening of symptoms, should be part of the counseling. Some clinicians prefer leuprolide because of the smaller needle size, while others prefer Goserelin. GnRHa treatment is administered for 3-4 months to shrink fibroids before myomectomy or hysterectomy, serving as a short-term preoperative therapy. This approach aims to avoid midline incisions, anemia, and the need for blood transfusions. Additionally, it can be used as a short-term treatment to prevent the need for surgery in women approaching menopause, particularly during late perimenopause, by reducing the bulk of fibroid and giving symptomatic relief.[3,4,8]

TABLE 2: Gonadotropin-releasing hormone (GnRH) agonist versus antagonist.	
GnRH agonist	**GnRH antagonist**
• It reduces estrogen and progesterone levels and blood flow to the fibroids to shrink them • It works by temporarily stopping the menstrual periods and causes menopausal state • Clinical evidence showed that up 30% reduction in fibroid size was achieved after 6 months of treatment • GnRHa also reduces blood loss and relieves pelvic pressure, urinary frequency, nocturia, and constipation • The most prescribed GnRHa is Zoladex which is injected either every monthly or 3 monthly and can be given up to 6 months maximum • The major side effect is severe bone thinning leading to osteoporosis. Other adverse effects include symptoms of menopause, i.e., hot flushes, headache, vaginal dryness, irregular bleeding, depression, hair loss, and musculoskeletal stiffness • *A temporary treatment only:* Once GnRHa treatment stops, the fibroids will return to their original size	• Reduction in fibroid size occurs more quickly compared to GnRHa agonist • Commonly, it is used preoperatively in young women and perimenopausal women, e.g., Cetrorelix • Side effects include hot flushes, amenorrhea • Normal periods return within 1 month of discontinuation of treatment • It is a short-term therapy only • Fibroid regrows after stopping the medication

The common side effects of GnRHa treatment include menopausal-like symptoms, such as hot flushes, increased sweating, and vaginal dryness. Additionally, red degeneration has been reported following GnRH analog treatment.[9,14]

Less common side effects may include bone loss, particularly trabecular bone loss when treatment is administered for longer than 6 months. These side effects often lead to high rates of discontinuation and preclude long-term use of GnRHa therapy. To mitigate bone loss, "add-back" therapy with medications such as tibolone or raloxifene may be prescribed, aiming to minimize or eliminate bone mineral loss when used long term.[3,8]

Advantages:
- Decreases menorrhagia, especially in perimenopausal patients, and corrects anemia
- Decreases uterine volume by 30% and fibroid volume by 35%
- Decreases vascularity and blood loss during myomectomy
- Facilitates hysteroscopic/laparoscopic surgery

Disadvantages:
- Significant bone loss after 6 months of therapy
- Other side effects, i.e., hot flushes, vaginal dryness, frontal headache, arthralgia, and myalgia; other menopausal side effects are due to hypoestrogenic state caused by it.
- GnRHa not recommended for >6 months without add-back therapy.

■ VARIOUS ADD-BACK THERAPIES

- Equine estrogen 0.3–0.625 mg from 1 to 25 days + MPA 10 mg from 16 to 25 days

- *Continuous regimen:* MPA 2.5 mg + equine estrogen 0.3–0.625 mg
- *Continuous regimen:* E2 0.5 mg + norethisterone acetate (NETA) 0.1 mg
- *Selective estrogen receptor modulator (SERM):* Tibolone/Raloxifene—risk of vasomotor symptoms and venous thromboembolism, respectively.

Following discontinuation, menses return in 4–8 weeks and uterus size returns to previous size in 4–6 months. Because of rapid rebound in symptoms and side effects, they are used selectively as preoperative therapy.

The effectiveness of add-back therapy given over 1 year has been evaluated in a Cochrane review, which analyzed 12 RCTs including 622 patients. The review found that the use of MPA did not demonstrate any discernible impact on bone mass (BM), although there was observed uterine enlargement. Conversely, tibolone administration resulted in a reduction in BM loss and an enhancement in QoL. Raloxifene exhibited no significant influence on QoL but proved beneficial in preserving BM, with inconclusive evidence regarding its effects on bleeding, uterine volume, or vasomotor symptoms. Estriol usage lacked sufficient studies to evaluate its impact on uterine size, bleeding, or vasomotor symptoms, although it showed potential in preventing BM loss. Ipriflavone use did not appear to affect vasomotor symptoms, although a solitary study reported decreased BM loss. Additionally, a study suggested that combining conjugated estrogens with GnRHa led to a more pronounced reduction in uterine volume. These findings shed light on the diverse effects of add-back therapies when employed alongside GnRHa therapy, offering valuable insights into their implications for BM, uterine size, bleeding, and vasomotor symptoms over a sustained treatment period.[15]

ROLE OF PREOPERATIVE MEDICAL THERAPY BEFORE SURGERY

In a recent Cochrane review encompassing analysis from 38 RCTs including 3,623 patients, significant findings emerged regarding the preoperative use of GnRHa. The review concluded that GnRHa administration before surgery led to notable reductions in both uterine and fibroid volume. Additionally, preoperative hemoglobin (Hb) levels were observed to increase, contributing to a decrease in blood loss during the operation. Moreover, its use led to reduced operation time and lower complication rates, particularly in cases involving hysterectomy.[16]

GONADOTROPIN-RELEASING HORMONE ANTAGONIST (TABLE 2)

Elagolix

Elagolix is a GnRH antagonist and is an effective treatment for dysmenorrhea, non-menstrual pelvic pain, and dyspareunia due to endometriosis.[17,18] In a three-pronged trial involving premenopausal women with myomas and HMB, Elagolix was evaluated. The study observed a significant reduction in MBL, with the highest dose-dependent reduction observed at Elagolix dose of 300 mg twice daily compared to placebo. The addition of add-back regimens further enhanced the reduction in MBL. However, adverse events associated with Elagolix were found to be dose-independent, ranging from 70.0 to 81.3%. Adverse event rates were comparatively lower with placebo and add-back regimens. Hot flushes emerged as the most common side effect across all groups. The authors concluded that Elagolix demonstrated efficacy in reducing HMB among women with fibroids, and the addition of low-dose add-back regimens notably mitigated the occurrence of hot flushes.[19-21]

In a double-blind RCT, multiple ascending doses of Elagolix including 150 mg once daily and 100, 200, 300, or 400 mg twice daily, along with a placebo, administered over a 21-day period, were administered to 45 healthy premenopausal women to investigate its pharmacokinetics and pharmacodynamics.[22] However, Elagolix is still not licensed for use in uterine fibroid. Immediate suppression of GnRH by daily s/c inj. Ganirelix clinically decreases fibroid volume by 29% within 3 weeks. The main adverse effects of all GnRH antagonists are hypoestrogenic symptoms, i.e., hot flushes **(Table 2)**.

■ DRUGS UNDER TRIAL (TABLE 3)

GnRH Receptor Blocker

Relugolix (TAK-385) is the fourth orally active gonadotropin-releasing hormone receptor (GnRHR) blocker characterized by high affinity and potent antagonistic activity. In studies conducted on mice, it demonstrated ability to reduce uterus weight to levels comparable to those seen after ovariectomy. Additionally, it also led to the downregulation of GnRHR mRNA expression in the pituitary gland following 4 weeks of administration.[23]

Antiprogesterone/Antiprogestins/SPRM

Several antiprogestins do not solely exert their effects through "pure" antiprogestin activity but rather function by suppressing the expression of the progesterone receptor (PR) gene. This mechanism of action contributes to their efficacy in modulating hormonal pathways and treating conditions influenced by progesterone signaling.[24]

Ulipristal Acetate

Ulipristal acetate (UPA) is a SPRM, formerly known as CDB-2914. UPA shares a chemical structure similar to that of mifepristone. Recent research indicates that UPA exerts inhibitory effects on various molecular targets involved in fibroid pathophysiology. Authors have suggested a multifaceted mechanism by which UPA modulates fibroid growth and associated molecular pathways.[25]

TABLE 3: Summary of undertrial medical therapies.

Medical therapy	Outcome on fibroid size	Outcome on HMB
GnRHR blocker: Relugolix (TAK-385)	Decreases uterine weight	Decrease
SPRM: Mifepristone (RU486)	Decreases uterine volume by 40%	Decrease (but small risk of endometrial hyperplasia)
SPRM: Asoprisnil	Decreases by 35–40%	Decrease
SERM: Ormeloxifene	Unknown	Decrease
Oral progestogen: Dienogest	Unknown	May decrease
GnRH antagonist: Ganirelix (subcutaneous injection)	Decreases by 30–40%	Decrease
Aromatase inhibitors: Anastrozole, Letrozole	Decrease	Decrease

(GnRHa: gonadotropin-releasing hormone agonist; GnRHR: gonadotropin-releasing hormone receptor; HMB: heavy menstrual bleeding; SERM: selective estrogen receptor modulator; SPRM: selective progesterone receptor modulator)

Multicenter clinical trials labeled "PEARL I–IV" have established the role of UPA in the medical management of myomas.[26] In clinical trials, UPA demonstrated efficacy when given at daily doses of 5 and 10 mg, leading to reductions in fibroid size and improvements in HMB by 42% and 98%, respectively. Additionally, UPA resulted in amenorrhea in 89% of women, a level comparable to that achieved by GnRHa like leuprolide acetate. While the 5 mg dose was slightly less effective than the 10 mg dose, with a 36% reduction in fibroid size and 75% amenorrhea rate, this difference was not statistically significant. Notably, UPA demonstrated faster symptomatic improvement compared to GnRHa, achieving results within 1 week of treatment versus 3 weeks. Moreover, it exhibited fewer side effects, with only a 10% risk of hot flushes versus 40% with GnRHa. Recommendations for UPA 5 mg use were based on the findings of three RCTs involving women of reproductive age with symptomatic fibroids of at least 3 cm in diameter, where no statistical difference in effectiveness was observed between the 5 and 10 mg doses.[27,28]

In 2012, ulipristal received a medical license across Europe for its use in treating fibroids. The National Institute for Health and Care Excellence (NICE) guideline on HMB recommended UPA for women with fibroids measuring 3 cm or more in diameter.

Additionally, a fourth trial investigated the effectiveness and safety of 12-week cycles of 5 or 10 mg UPA daily in 451 women. The authors observed that 80% of subjects experienced control of excessive bleeding, with a mean reduction in fibroid volume of 54% and 58% for 5 and 10 mg, respectively. Furthermore, there was improvement in pain symptoms and overall QoL.[29] So 5 mg UPA was recommended for up to 4 courses for 3 months each. It was recommended to be used for unmarried girls and perimenopausal women to avoid surgery and it was reported that it had no effect on BMD.

A systematic meta-analysis examining the effects of UPA in women with fibroids encompassed four RCTs. Among these, three compared the drug with a placebo, while one compared it with GnRHa for symptomatic relief. The trials consistently reported improvements in HMB, demonstrated by the significant achievement of amenorrhea ($p = 0.00001$), along with enhancements in QoL parameters and reductions in fibroid size.[30]

Similarly, a study reported that UPA was effective in reducing fibroid volume, pain, and bleeding and in markedly improving QoL, even during the off-treatment intervals. No significant changes in laboratory parameters were observed, documenting the effectiveness of UPA as an alternative to surgery.[31]

Wagenfeld and colleagues similarly concluded in their review that UPA represents a valuable option in preventing hysterectomy by giving patients an option of suitable effective long-term medical treatment.[24]

Later Cochrane review confirmed the occurrence of progesterone receptor modulator-associated endometrial changes (PAEC)[32] and suggested trying a mixed regimen using first a GnRHa to get an inactive endometrium and then beginning treatment with SPRM.[33] A previous study on the safety of UPA had also concluded that it induced endometrial changes, which were both benign and reversible.[34]

Following reports of a rare serious liver injury, i.e., liver failure, the European Medicines Agency (EMA) Pharmacovigilance Risk Assessment Committee (PRAC) carried out a full evaluation. They concluded that UPA may be responsible for the liver failure and is contraindicated in liver damage and hence advocated liver function tests at various points during treatment.[35] Later in 2018, it was recommended that it should be given preoperatively for four courses, lasting up to 3 months, with measurement of liver function before the start of treatment, monthly for the first 2 courses and once before each new treatment course.[35]

However, later, there were reported cases of severe liver injury associated with UPA, leading to liver transplant. As a result, the Medicines and Healthcare products Regulatory Agency (MHRA) suspended the license for UPA in March 2020, and the National Institute for Health and Care Excellence (NICE) guidelines on its use were temporarily withdrawn.

The MHRA reinstated that UPA is indicated only for intermittent treatment of uterine fibroids >3 cm diameter, which were symptomatic before menopause in patients either not suitable, declined, or with failed surgical procedures, i.e., UAE, which is a better option.[4] Ulipristal 5 mg up to four courses should be given to premenopausal women with HMB with fibroid >3 cm and with no liver injury and in whom UAE is unsuitable or has failed.[36]

The EMA's committee for medicinal products for human use recommended marketing authorization for UPA in the preoperative treatment of uterine myomas.[37]

Mifepristone (RU486)

Mifepristone is indeed a SPRM, which when administered orally at doses of 25–50 mg daily for 3 months or at 5 mg daily for 5–6 months has shown a significant decrease in symptom severity and an increase in QoL questionnaire scores. Mifepristone has been observed to decrease mean uterine volume by 48% after 6 months of treatment. However, it may also lead to endometrial hyperplasia. Major side effects associated with mifepristone include headache, nausea, mood swings, diarrhea, decreased libido, weakness, fatigue, hot flushes, endometrial hyperplasia, and increased liver enzymes.[38] Arora et al. reported that weekly or biweekly doses of 50 mg of mifepristone were effective.[39] In a previous study, 10 mg daily of mifepristone was used by the vaginal route, with significant reduction in the volume of fibroids.[40]

Asoprisnil

Asoprisnil is also a SPRM administered in doses of 5–25 mg daily and leads to dose-dependent reduction in uterine bleeding. In 25 mg daily dose, approximately 70% of women achieved amenorrhea. Common side effects include bloating, flatulence, breast pain, hot flushes, and night sweats. Asymptomatic ovarian cysts have also been reported with it.

Ormeloxifene

Ormeloxifene is a SERM. Dose is 60 mg twice a week for 3 months followed by 60 mg once a week for 3 months and it decreases MBL.

Aromatase Inhibitor

Anastrozole

Anastrozole is an aromatase inhibitor, which has shown efficacy in reducing the volume of fibroids when administered orally at a dose of 1 mg daily for 3 months. In a trial involving 20 patients, it was observed that anastrozole led to an average reduction in fibroid volume of 9.32%, with some patients experiencing reductions of up to 32%.[41]

Letrozole

Letrozole, an aromatase inhibitor primarily licensed for use in breast cancer treatment, has shown promise in the management of uterine fibroids. Clinical trial data indicate that when administered orally at a dose of 5 mg daily for 3 months, it resulted in a reduction in the size of fibroids and improvement in symptoms of HMB, without adversely affecting BMD. In a study involving 70 patients with fibroids >5 cm, treatment with letrozole at a dose of 2.5 mg daily for 12 weeks led to a notable 45.6% reduction in fibroid volume.[42]

Danazol

Danazol is given in a dose of 200–400 mg tds for 3 months. It is not recommended due to androgenic side effects.

Gestrinone

Gestrinone has antiestrogenic and anti-progesterone effect but antiandrogenic side effect. Dose is 2.5 mg twice a week.

NEWER DRUGS

Relugolix–estradiol–norethisterone Acetate

A combination therapy available in tablet form at doses of 40–1–0.5 mg, respectively, addresses the pressing need for effective management of symptoms associated with uterine fibroids. It is recommended as a viable option for treating moderate-to-severe symptoms of uterine fibroids in women of reproductive age. Offering potential cost benefits, this treatment stands out for several reasons: It provides an effective nonsurgical approach, administered orally for convenience; unlike GnRHa, it imposes no restrictions on treatment duration and importantly it is well tolerated while preserving the uterus.[1]

Combination therapy is comparable to GnRHa as both are treatment options in moderate-to-severe bleeding but later can be used only for 6 months. The clinical data supporting its efficacy stemmed from two identical phase III RCTs, LIBERTY 1 and LIBERTY 2, which suggested that this combination therapy is likely to be as effective as GnRHa while being well tolerated with reduction in symptoms with sustained treatment effectiveness being observed over a 2-year period.[1]

OBE-2109

It is fifth nonpeptide inhibitor (code-named OBE-2109) which can be used in dose of 100–200 mg to induce amenorrhea.[43]

CONCLUSION

Scientifically validated medical management of fibroid has been available for the past 40 years now. First-line medical therapy is NSAID and tranexamic acid, which do not decrease fibroid size. GnRHa and ulipristal should be used judiciously, only in symptomatic perimenopausal women or preoperatively to reduce the size of the fibroid. The most promising medical treatments for fibroid till date belong to two categories of drugs that are SPRM and orally active GnRHR blockers. Nonsurgical options such as UAE are preferred over ulipristal because of the risk of liver failure.

REFERENCES

1. Syed YY. Relugolix/Estradiol/Norethisterone (Norethindrone) Acetate: A review in symptomatic uterine fibroids. Drugs. 2022;82(15):1549-56.
2. Spies JB. Current role of uterine artery embolization in the management of uterine fibroids. Clin Obstet Gynecol. 2016;59(1):93-102.
3. Singh SS, Belland L. Contemporary management of uterine fibroids: focus on emerging medical treatments. Curr Med Res Opin. 2015;31(1):1-12.
4. NICE. Heavy menstrual bleeding: Assessment and management. London: National Institute for Health and Care Excellence; 2021.

5. Donnez J, Donnez O, Dolmans MM. With the advent of selective progesterone receptor modulators, what is the place of myoma surgery in current practice? Fertil Steril. 2014;102(3):640-8.
6. Gurusamy KS, Vaughan J, Fraser IS, Best LMJ, Richards T. Medical therapies for uterine fibroids—A systematic review and network meta-analysis of randomised controlled trials. PLoS One. 2016;11(2):e0149631.
7. Bartels CB, Cayton KC, Chuong FS, Holthouser K, Arian SE, Abraham T, et al. An Evidence-based approach to the medical management of fibroids: A systematic review. Clin Obstet Gynecol. 2016;59(1):30-52.
8. Maybin JA, Critchley HO. Medical management of heavy menstrual bleeding. Womens Health (Lond). 2016;12(1):27-34.
9. Bitzer J, Heikinheimo O, Nelson AL, Calaf-Alsina J, Fraser IS. Medical management of heavy menstrual bleeding: A comprehensive review of the literature. Obstet Gynecol Surv. 2015;70(2):115-30.
10. Sriprasert I, Pakrashi T, Kimble T, Archer DF. Heavy menstrual bleeding diagnosis and medical management. Contracept Reprod Med. 2017;2:20.
11. Fox KE. Management of heavy menstrual bleeding in general practice. Curr Med Res Opin. 2012;28(9):1517-25.
12. Kaunitz AM, Inki P. The levonorgestrel-releasing intrauterine system in heavy menstrual bleeding: A benefit-risk review. Drugs. 2012;72(2):193-215.
13. Endrikat J, Vilos G, Muysers C, Fortier M, Solomayer E, Lukkari-Lax E. The levonorgestrel-releasing intrauterine system provides a reliable, long-term treatment option for women with idiopathic menorrhagia. Arch Gynecol Obstet. 2012; 285(1):117-21.
14. Hachiya K, Kato H, Kawaguchi S, Kojima T, Nishikawa Y, Fujiwara S, et al. Red degeneration of a uterine fibroid following the administration of gonadotropin releasing hormone agonists. J Obstet Gynaecol. 2016; 36(8):1018-9.
15. Moroni RM, Martins WP, Ferriani RA, Vieira CS, Nastri CO, Candido Dos Reis FJ, et al. Add-back therapy with GnRH analogues for uterine fibroids. Cochrane Database Syst Rev. 2015;2015(3):CD010854.
16. Lethaby A, Puscasiu L, Vollenhoven B. Preoperative medical therapy before surgery for uterine fibroids. Cochrane Database Syst Rev. 2017;11(11):CD000547.
17. Taylor HS, Giudice LC, Lessey BA, Abrao MS, Kotarski J, Archer DF, et al. Treatment of endometriosis-associated pain with Elagolix, an Oral GnRH antagonist. N Engl J Med. 2017;377(1):28-40.
18. Surrey E, Taylor HS, Giudice L, Lessey BA, Abrao MS, Archer DF, et al. Long-term outcomes of Elagolix in women with endometriosis: Results from two extension studies. Obstet Gynecol. 2018;132(1):147-60.
19. Kim SM, Yoo T, Lee SY, Kim EJ, Lee SM, Lee MH, et al. Effect of SKI2670, a novel, orally active, non-peptide GnRH antagonist, on hypothalamic-pituitary-gonadal axis. Life Sci. 2015;139:166-74.
20. Kim SM, Lee M, Lee SY, Park E, Lee SM, Kim EJ, et al. Discovery of an orally bioavailable gonadotropin-releasing hormone receptor antagonist. J Med Chem. 2016;59(19):9150-72.
21. Archer DF, Stewart EA, Jain RI, Feldman RA, Lukes AS, North JD, et al. Elagolix for the management of heavy menstrual bleeding associated with uterine fibroids: Results from a phase 2a proof-of-concept study. Fertil Steril. 2017;108(1):152-60.e4.
22. Ng J, Chwalisz K, Carter DC, Klein CE. Dose-dependent suppression of gonadotropins and ovarian hormones by Elagolix in healthy premenopausal women. J Clin Endocrinol Metab. 2017;102(5):1683-91.
23. Nakata D, Masaki T, Tanaka A, Yoshimatsu M, Akinaga Y, Asada M, et al. Suppression of the hypothalamic-pituitary-gonadal axis by TAK-385 (relugolix), a novel, investigational, orally active, small molecule gonadotropin-releasing hormone (GnRH) antagonist: Studies in human GnRH receptor knock-in mice. Eur J Pharmacol. 2014;723:167-74.
24. Wagenfeld A, Saunders PT, Whitaker L, Critchley HOD. Selective progesterone receptor modulators (SPRMs): Progesterone receptor action, mode of action on the

24. endometrium and treatment options in gynecological therapies. Expert Opin Ther Targets. 2016;20(9):1045-54.
25. Ciarmela P, Carrarelli P, Islam MS, Janjusevic M, Zupi E, Tosti C, et al. Ulipristal acetate modulates the expression and functions of activin a in leiomyoma cells. Reprod Sci. 2014;21(9):1120-5.
26. Powell M, Dutta D. Esmya® and the PEARL studies: a review. Womens Health (Lond). 2016;12(6):544-8.
27. Donnez J, Tomaszewski J, Vázquez F, Bouchard P, Lemieszczuk B, Baró F, et al.; PEARL II Study Group. Ulipristal acetate versus leuprolide acetate for uterine fibroids. N Engl J Med. 2012;366(5):421-32.
28. Donnez J, Tomaszewski J, Vázquez F, Bouchard P, Lemieszczuk B, Baró F, et al. Ulipristal acetate versus placebo for fibroid treatment before surgery. N Engl J Med. 2012;366(5):409-20.
29. Donnez J, Hudecek R, Donnez O, Matule D, Arhendt HJ, Zatik J, et al. Efficacy and safety of repeated use of ulipristal acetate in uterine fibroids. Fertil Steril. 2015;103(2):519-27.e3.
30. Kalampokas T, Kamath M, Boutas I, Kalampokas E. Ulipristal acetate for uterine fibroids: A systematic review and meta-analysis. Gynecol Endocrinol. 2016; 32(2):91-6.
31. Donnez J, Donnez O, Matule D, Ahrendt HJ, Hudecek R, Zatik J, et al. Long-term medical management of uterine fibroids with ulipristal acetate. Fertil Steril. 2016;105(1):165-73.e4.
32. Milliano ID, Hattum DV, Ket JCF, Huirne JAF, Hehenkamp WJK. Endometrial changes during ulipristal acetate use: a systematic review. Eur J Obstet Gynecol Reprod Biol. 2017;214:56-64.
33. Fauser BC, Donnez J, Bouchard P, Barlow DH, Vázquez F, Arriagada P, et al. Safety after extended repeated use of ulipristal acetate for uterine fibroids. PLoS One. 2017; 12(3):e0173523.
34. Donnez J, Donnez O, Dolmans MM. Safety of treatment of uterine fibroids with the selective progesterone receptor modulator, ulipristal acetate. Expert Opin Drug Saf. 2016;15(12):1679-86.
35. European Medicines Agency. Esmya: New measures to minimise risk of rare but serious liver injury. [online] Available from www.ema.europa.eu/ema/index.jsp?curl=pages/medicines/human/referrals/Esmya/human_referral_prac_000070.jsp&mid=WC0b01ac05805c516f [Last accessed July, 2024].
36. Murji A, Whitaker L, Chow TL, Sobel ML. Selective progesterone receptor modulators (SPRMs) for uterine fibroids. Cochrane Database Syst Rev. 2017;4(4):CD010770.
37. Farris M, Bastianelli C, Rosato E, Brosens I, Benagiano G. Uterine fibroids: an update on current and emerging medical treatment options. Ther Clin Risk Manag. 2019;15:157-78.
38. Kapur A, Angomchanu R, Dey M. Efficacy of use of long-term, low-dose mifepristone for the treatment of fibroids. J Obstet Gynaecol India. 2016;66(Suppl 1):494-8.
39. Arora D, Chawla J, Kochar SPS, Sharma JC. A randomized control trial to assess efficacy of mifepristone in medical management of uterine fibroid. Med J Armed Forces India. 2017;73(3):267-73.
40. Yerushalmi GM, Gilboa Y, Jakobson-Setton A, Tadir Y, Goldchmit C, Katz D, et al. Vaginal mifepristone for the treatment of symptomatic uterine leiomyomata: an open-label study. Fertil Steril. 2014;101(2):496-500.
41. Hilário SG, Bozzini N, Borsari R, Baracat E. Action of aromatase inhibitor for treatment of uterine leiomyoma in perimenopausal patients. Fertil Steril. 2009;91(1):240-3.
42. Mohammad EP, Mina A, Saeed A, Rajaeefard A, Zarei A, Kazerooni T, et al. A randomized, controlled clinical trial comparing the effects of aromatase inhibitor (letrozole) and gonadotropin-releasing hormone agonist (triptorelin) on uterine leiomyoma volume and hormonal status. Fertility Sterility. 2010;93(1):192-8.
43. Pohl O, Marchand L, Fawkes N, Gotteland JP, Loumaye E. Gonadotropin-releasing hormone receptor antagonist mono- and combination therapy with estradiol/norethindrone acetate add-back: pharmacodynamics and safety of OBE2109. J Clin Endocrinol Metab. 2018;103(2):497-504.

CHAPTER 8

Presurgical Hormonal Treatment

Vijay Chandrakant Pawar

■ INTRODUCTION

The presurgical treatment of fibroids includes gonadotropin-releasing hormone (GnRH) analogs, progestins, selective estrogen receptor modulators (SERM), selective progesterone receptor modulators (SPRM), and dopamine agonists.

It has been well known since a long time that the fibroids have estrogen and progesterone receptors (PRs) and the hormonal cycle influences the growth of the fibroids. So, by manipulating these hormones, one can decrease the size and growth of the fibroids.

■ INDICATIONS FOR PRETREATMENT

- Patients with severe anemia waiting for hysterectomy
- To reduce blood loss during the surgery
- To reduce the size of the fibroids before surgery, especially in difficult cases
- Prior to myomectomy, it can be used to reduce the size of the fibroid and reduce the overall complications of the surgery.

■ GONADOTROPIN-RELEASING HORMONE AGONISTS

Synthetic long-acting GnRH agonists such as leuprolide acetate depot 3.75 mg intramuscular monthly can be used.

Mechanism of Action

Flare effect followed by suppression and causing pseudomenopause: They initially increase follicle stimulating hormone (FSH) and luteinizing hormone (LH) secretion. After that, they subsequently cause receptor downregulation, followed 1–3 weeks later by a hypogonadotropic hypogonadal state, often termed—"pseudomenopause". This hypoestrogenic state contributes to the pharmacologic efficacy of GnRH agonists, as fibroids' growth is stimulated by estrogen.[1-3]

There is correction of anemia as blood loss during menses decreases as the uterine volume reduces.

Since the patient's anemia is corrected, the patient's recovery in the postoperative period gets improved and hence the duration of hospital stay reduces.

However, it is associated with histological changes in uterine fibroids that may complicate surgical intervention. Because of myoma degeneration and loss of space between the fibroid and myoma, enucleation becomes difficult.

Small fibroids may become difficult to identify as they become soft and hence can be missed during laparoscopic myomectomy.

The use of preoperative lupride depot in hysteroscopic resection of submucosal fibroids helps in reducing the operative time. So, this ultimately reduces the fluid absorption and makes difficult procedures easy.

GnRH Add-back Therapy

Long-term GnRH therapy causes a hypoestrogenic state and leads to menopausal symptoms such as decreased bone mineral density (BMD), atrophic vaginitis, and hot flushes. This necessitates the use of hormonal add-back therapy to offset these issues if they are considered to be used for a long term.

GnRH Antagonists

Gonadotropin-releasing hormone antagonists cause immediate fall in LH and FSH levels and have no initial flare effect so they can be used for preoperative treatment of fibroids like the agonist; however, the current drawback is nonavailability of long-acting preparations. Currently, if one chooses to give an antagonist, it has to be given daily for few months before some changes can be observed. Injection Ganirelix 2 mg SC daily for 1–3 months results in rapid reduction of leiomyoma and uterine volume in premenopausal women with minor side effects. If longer-acting GnRH antagonists become available, pretreatment with GnRH antagonist should be preferred over GnRH agonists prior to surgery.[4]

SELECTIVE PROGESTERONE RECEPTOR MODULATORS

Selective progesterone receptor modulators have tissue-specific effects at PRs, and they can have either a complete PR agonist or an antagonist profile or a mixed agonist/antagonist profile. Mifepristone and ulipristal have emerged as a promising therapy for the management of uterine fibroids.[5]

Mifepristone

Long-term administration of low-dose mifepristone for a year in a dose of 5–10 mg/day orally results in myoma shrinkage and amelioration of symptoms. However, there is a slight increase in the rate of low-grade endometrial hyperplasia, but no evidence of premalignant potential.

Ulipristal

The PEARL trial phases 1–4 have proved that ulipristal 5–10 mg daily for 12 weeks significantly helps in symptomatic relief and volume reduction of fibroids. However, because of its liver toxicity issues, it is currently not recommended.[2,5]

SELECTIVE ESTROGEN RECEPTOR MODULATORS—TAMOXIFEN

Tamoxifen 20 mg daily for 6 months reduces the amount of bleeding but no change in the size of the fibroid. However, it has agonist action on the endometrium leading to endometrial hyperplasia. The other side effects like hot flushes and dizziness along with endometrial hyperplasia make this drug a poor choice for treatment of fibroids.[2,6]

Aromatase Inhibitor

Aromatase inhibitors are equally effective as compared to GnRH agonists in the medical management of fibroids. They reduce the size and have less side effects like hot flushes, compared to GnRH agonists over a period of 12 weeks.[2,7]

Letrozole (2.5 mg OD × 12 weeks) and Anastrozole (1 mg × 12 weeks) can be used in the treatment of fibroids. They reduce the aromatase levels in the fibroid, thus reducing the local levels of estrogen. This causes shrinking of fibroids.

Progestins

Recently, Dienogest has been advocated to be used in the treatment of fibroids. However, further studies are required to advocate its use in fibroids. It is not recommended for preoperative treatment of fibroids.[8]

Levonorgestrel Intrauterine System

Levonorgestrel intrauterine system (LNG IUS) reduces uterine bleeding but has very less effect on the size of the fibroid. Hence, it is not recommended for preoperative treatment to reduce the size of the fibroid. However, it can be used to reduce the amount of bleeding and correction of anemia before the patient is awaiting surgery.[2]

ORAL CONTRACEPTIVE PILLS

Combination oral contraceptives (COCs) were considered a risk factor for fibroid growth in the past, as they stimulate the growth of fibroids. However, a recent meta-analysis suggests that they reduce the bleeding associated with fibroids as it suppresses the endometrium but does not have any effect on the size of the fibroid. However, it will not be prudent to use OC pills prior to planned surgery so they are not recommended preoperatively.[2]

DOPAMINE AGONIST—CABERGOLINE

One of the effective hormones on myoma growth is prolactin which is secreted in both pituitary and uterine cells and can act on the myometrium as a growth hormone in the form of autocrine and paracrine. Regarding this effect, prolactin-lowering agents, like dopamine agonists, can inhibit the growth of myoma and improve the symptoms. Using this principle, 0.5 mg of cabergoline orally once a week for 3 months can be used. It reduces the size of the fibroid, improves the hemoglobin, and reduces the blood loss.[9]

CONCLUSION

The main role of preoperative hormonal treatment in fibroids is to reduce the size, improve the anemia, and reduce the blood loss. GnRH agonist, LNG IUS, and aromatase inhibitor are the main choices in the preoperative management of fibroids awaiting surgery.

REFERENCES

1. American College of Obstetricians and Gynecologists. ACOG practice bulletin. Alternatives to hysterectomy in the management of leiomyomas. Obstet Gynecol. 2008; 112:387-400.
2. Sohn GS, Cho S, Kim YM, Cho CH, Kim MR, Lee SR; Working Group of Society of Uterine Leiomyoma. Current medical treatment of uterine fibroids. Obstet Gynecol Sci. 2018;61(2):192-201.
3. Lethaby A, Vollenhoven B, Sowter M. Preoperative GnRH analogue therapy before hysterectomy or myomectomy for uterine fibroids. Cochrane Database Syst Rev. 2000;CD000547.
4. Flierman PA, Oberyé JJ, van der Hulst VP, de Blok S. Rapid reduction of leiomyoma volume during treatment with the GnRH antagonist ganirelix. BJOG. 2005;112:638-42.
5. Maruo T. Progesterone and progesterone receptor modulator in uterine leiomyoma growth. Gynecol Endocrinol. 2007;23:186-7.
6. Wu T, Chen X, Xie L. Selective estrogen receptor modulators (SERMs) for uterine leiomyomas. Cochrane Database Syst Rev. 2007;CD005287.
7. Song H, Lu D, Navaratnam K, Shi G. Aromatase inhibitors for uterine fibroids. Cochrane Database Syst Rev. 2013;CD009505
8. Ichigo S, Takagi H, Matsunami K, Suzuki N, Imai A. Beneficial effects of dienogest on uterine myoma volume: a retrospective controlled study comparing with gonadotropin-releasing hormone agonist. Arch Gynecol Obstet. 2011;284:667-70.
9. Vahdat M, Kashanian M, Ghaziani N, Sheikhansari N. Evaluation of the effects of cabergoline (Dostinex) on women with symptomatic myomatous uterus: a randomized trial. Eur J Obstet Gynecol Reprod Biol. 2016;206:74-8.

CHAPTER 9

Laparoscopic Myomectomy

Parul Sinha

■ INTRODUCTION

Uterine fibroids (leiomyomas or myomas) are the most common type of pelvic tumor in women. Uterine fibroids, medically known as leiomyomas or myomas, are extremely common, affecting a significant portion of women during their reproductive years. In fact, research suggests that up to 70–80% of women may develop fibroids by the age of 50 years.

These tumors can vary in size, number, and location within the uterus, leading to a wide range of symptoms and health complications. The impact of uterine fibroids on women's health can be substantial, often causing symptoms such as heavy menstrual bleeding, pelvic pain, pressure on the bladder or bowel, and reproductive issues including infertility or recurrent miscarriages. Additionally, fibroids can negatively affect a woman's quality of life, leading to physical discomfort, emotional distress, and limitations in daily activities.

Given the prevalence and potential impact of uterine fibroids on women's health and well-being, discussing treatment options becomes crucial. By understanding the available interventions and their respective benefits and risks, women and their healthcare providers can make informed decisions tailored to individual needs and preferences. Therefore, exploring various treatment modalities, ranging from conservative management to surgical interventions, is essential in addressing the multifaceted nature of uterine fibroids and optimizing patient outcomes.

The various modalities of treatment include expectant management, medical therapy, conservative procedures like endometrial ablation, uterine artery embolization, magnetic resonance guided focused ultrasound, and surgical options of myomectomy, radiofrequency ablation (RFA), and hysterectomy. Myomectomy involves the surgical removal of leiomyomas from the uterus. This can be accomplished using an open abdominal, laparoscopic, hysteroscopic, or vaginal approach. Other laparoscopic procedures, including uterine artery occlusion and myolysis, are infrequently used. In the following text, we review laparoscopic myomectomy and other laparoscopic procedures for the treatment of uterine leiomyomas.

■ INDICATIONS

- Laparoscopic myomectomy is done in patients with symptomatic intramural or subserosal leiomyomas where future childbearing is required **(Fig. 1)**.
- Fibroid mapping which assesses the location, size, and number of leiomyomas

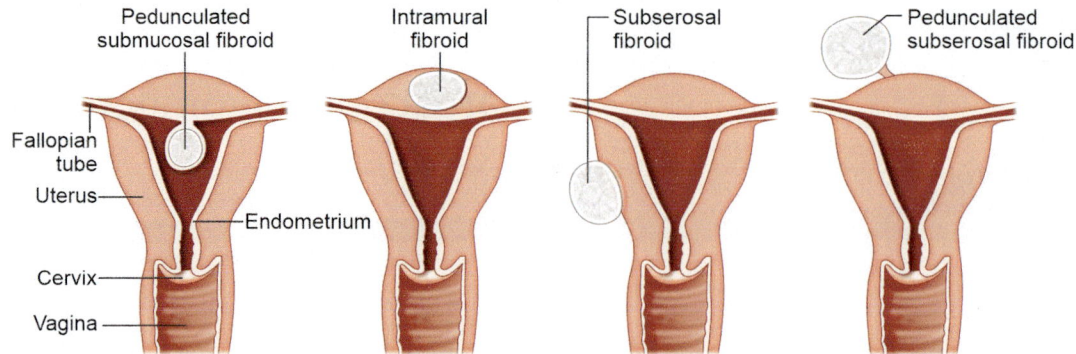

Fig. 1: Patients with symptomatic intramural or subserosal leiomyomas where future childbearing is required.

guides the choice for open versus laparoscopic route of surgery and also takes into consideration the surgical expertise (e.g., skill of laparoscopic suturing).[1]

- *Surgical expertise:* Under the discussion of surgical expertise, it is important to clarify "laparoscopic suturing" and emphasize its significance in ensuring effective closure of uterine defects. Laparoscopic suturing refers to the delicate skill of stitching tissue together using specialized instruments inserted through small incisions during minimally invasive surgery. Proficient suturing skills are crucial in laparoscopic myomectomy for meticulously closing any incisions made in the uterus to remove fibroids. Effective closure not only helps prevent excessive bleeding during the procedure but also reduces the risk of postoperative complications such as infection and uterine rupture. Routine preoperative use of gonadotropin-releasing hormone (GnRH) agonists is not advocated.

CONTRAINDICATIONS

In patients with medical comorbidities and in cervical and uterine cancers, laparoscopy and uterine conservation are contraindicated.

PREOPERATIVE EVALUATION AND PREPARATION

- Information and counseling of the patient and attendants about other available treatment options such as medical and interventional radiology should be done.
- They should be explained about the various complications of the procedure, including preoperative consents for conversion to laparotomy if needed and the chances of recurrence of fibroid-associated symptoms.
- The advantages and disadvantages of power morcellation and the remote risk of spread of malignant cells in an unsuspected uterine malignancy should be explained to the patient.
- Finally, the procedure that is most appropriate for them should be selected on the basis of shared decision-making.
- Imaging methods like pelvic ultrasonography or magnetic resonance imaging (MRI) should be used to confirm the presence of uterine leiomyomas, doing fibroid mapping by assessing their approximate number and location and identifying coincidental lesions like ovarian cysts, which, if present, may impact surgical planning.

- MRI has proven to be more accurate in assessing myoma size, number, and location.[2,3] It also has an upper edge in diagnosing adenomyosis which can present like leiomyomas making myomectomy more difficult.
- The use of prophylactic antibiotics prior to laparoscopic myomectomy varies according to the surgeon's choice, given in patients in whom there are chances of unexpected entry into the uterine cavity based on imaging, anticipation of a prolonged operating time, or increased blood loss and in patients with comorbid conditions like obesity and diabetes. The American College of Obstetricians and Gynecologists (ACOG) does not recommend the administration of prophylactic antibiotics for laparoscopic procedures in which the bowel or vagina is not entered.[4]

Prophylactic Antibiotics

The statement about prophylactic antibiotics may deviate from the recommendation of the ACOG, so it is essential to address this discrepancy and provide reasoning for the surgeon's choice if it differs from the ACOG recommendation. While ACOG advises against routine use of prophylactic antibiotics for laparoscopic procedures not involving the bowel or vagina, individual surgeon preferences and patient-specific factors may influence the decision to administer prophylactic antibiotics. Factors such as the anticipated operating time, potential blood loss, and patient comorbidities, as well as the possibility of inadvertently entering the uterine cavity despite preoperative imaging, should be considered in the decision-making process. It is important for surgeons to weigh the risks and benefits on a case-by-case basis and adhere to best practices while considering patient safety. However, even with preoperative imaging it may be difficult to predict which patients will require entry into the uterine cavity.

Thromboprophylaxis

Patients undergoing laparoscopic myomectomy require appropriate thromboprophylaxis because they are at low risk for venous thromboembolism (duration >45 minutes; *Caprini risk score:* 2 points).

■ PROCEDURE

- *Port placement:* The site of port placement is determined by the position and size of the myomas to be removed and is usually higher than the fundus of the uterus to allow access to the myomas. If the uterus lies near or above the level of the umbilicus, a left upper quadrant approach may be used.[5]
- *Initial survey:* The camera is inserted following initial port placement, and a survey of the entire pelvis and abdomen is done. In case of extensive adhesive disease or other unexpected findings, the procedure is converted to laparotomy.
- *Port size and placement:* These may also vary depending on the surgeon's preference. Two ports of sizes 12 and 5 mm are placed on either the patient's right side (for right-handed surgeons) or the patient's left side (for left-handed surgeons) with a 5-mm port on the contralateral side.
- *Myometrial incision and myoma dissection:* 10 mL of vasopressin (20 units dissolved in 100 mL saline) are injected into the myometrium overlying each fibroid. This is followed by a transverse myometrial incision directly over the

myoma, which is deepened until reaching a definite myoma tissue and the avascular plane just deep to the capsule of the myoma **(Fig. 2)**. Each myoma is then grasped with a tenaculum for traction, and using blunt and sharp (electrosurgical or ultrasonic) dissection, the plane between the myometrium and myoma is identified, and the myomas are separated one by one **(Fig. 3)**.

- *Control of bleeding:* Bleeding from large vessels at the site from where the myoma is separated is controlled by desiccating briefly with bipolar electrosurgical paddles. Excessive desiccation should be avoided as it devascularizes the myometrium, increasing the risk of uterine rupture in subsequent pregnancies.
- *Morcellation if needed:* In case of difficulty in removing the myomas through the existing ports, morcellation of the myoma (with or without an in-bag containment system) can be done.
- *Closure of uterine defects:* During closure of uterine defects, meticulous attention to detail is essential to prevent complications such as uterine rupture in future pregnancies.[6]
- *Closure of uterine defects:* The uterine defects can then be closed with delayed absorbable sutures in one, two, or three layers, depending on the depth of the defect. Meticulous closure of the defects is crucial to ensure proper healing and reduce the risk of complications.
- *Identification of uterine cavity entry:* To identify entrance into the uterine cavity, methylene blue dye may be placed into the cavity via a transcervical catheter. This dye can be observed if the cavity is entered during the procedure. All defects, including serosa, should be closed, and the principles of open abdominal myomectomy must be adhered to as far as feasible **(Fig. 4)**.
- *Irrigation and adhesion prevention:* The pelvis and abdomen are irrigated with normal saline, and the fluid is suctioned to maintain a clear surgical field. Effective measures for preventing adhesion formation are employed **(Fig. 5)**, although their safety and effectiveness have not been definitively established. Adhesion barriers or antiadhesion agents may be utilized based on surgeon's preference and institutional protocols.

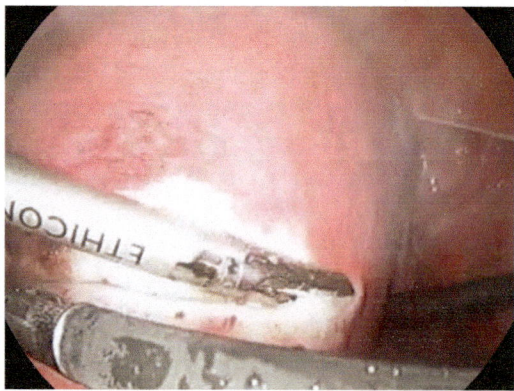

Fig. 2: Transverse myometrial incision over the myoma.

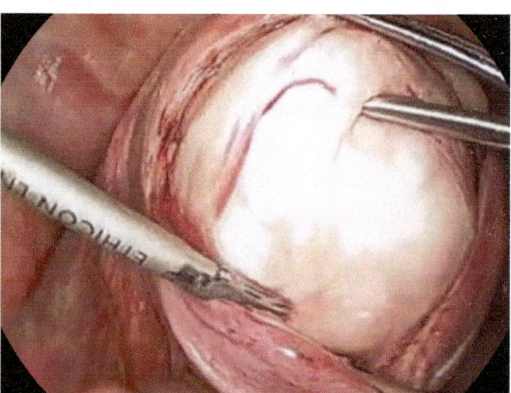

Fig. 3: Myoma separation after grasping with a tenaculum.

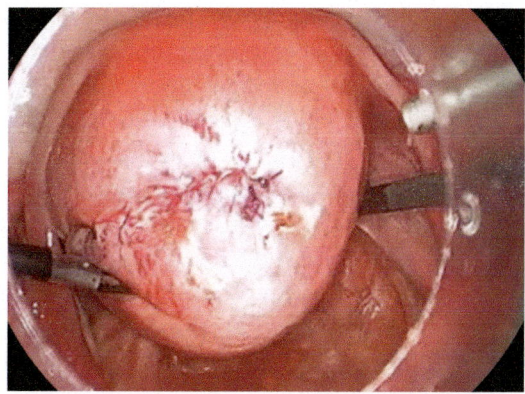

Fig. 4: Identification of uterine cavity entry.

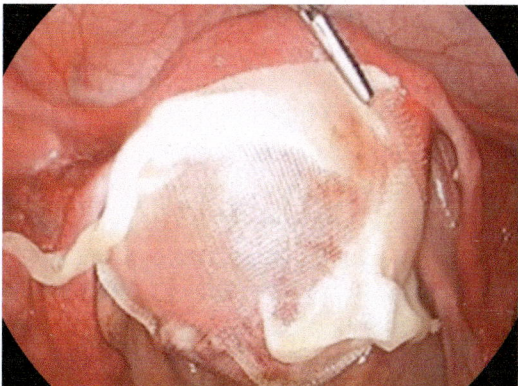

Fig. 5: Measures for preventing adhesion formation.

COMPLICATIONS

- Laparoscopic and open abdominal myomectomy have demonstrated similar complication rates, but laparoscopic myomectomy typically results in lower overall morbidity and a shorter recovery time compared to open myomectomy.
- Major complications, such as bleeding requiring blood transfusion, visceral injury, and procedural failure, have been associated with specific leiomyoma characteristics. These include size >5 cm, removal of more than three myomas, and intraligamentous location.[7]
- Rates of hemorrhage and blood transfusion during myomectomy procedures have been reported to range from 0.1% to 6%. The average reported blood loss varies from 80 to 248 mL, with a wide range of reported values (20–2,000 mL).[8,9]
- Conversion from laparoscopic myomectomy to laparotomy may be necessary if initial evaluation reveals any pathology that does not favor a laparoscopic approach, such as dense adhesions or malignancy. Additionally, conversion to laparotomy may be required to manage intraoperative complications, such as significant hemorrhage.

FUTURE PREGNANCY

- Patients with significant uterine disruption should wait 3–6 months before attempting to conceive,[10] allowing adequate time for the uterus to heal following myomectomy.
- Both open abdominal and laparoscopic myomectomy procedures may result in an increased risk of uterine rupture during future pregnancies. This risk arises due to the surgical incisions made in the uterus during the removal of fibroids, which can weaken the uterine wall.
- Many experts advise cesarean delivery as a conservative approach in most patients who have undergone myomectomy. Cesarean delivery is recommended to minimize the risk of uterine rupture during labor, particularly in patients who have had extensive myomectomies or multiple fibroids removed.
- The increased risk of uterine rupture after myomectomy is well documented in the literature. Studies have shown that the risk of uterine rupture during subsequent pregnancies is higher in women who have undergone myomectomy compared to

those who have not. Factors such as the size and location of the fibroids removed, the number of fibroids removed, and the type of myomectomy procedure performed can influence the risk of uterine rupture.
- While the absolute risk of uterine rupture after myomectomy is relatively low, it is important for patients and healthcare providers to be aware of this potential complication. Close monitoring during pregnancy and delivery, along with careful consideration of the mode of delivery, is essential in managing the risk of uterine rupture in women who have undergone myomectomy.
- Further research and long-term follow-up studies are needed to better understand the factors contributing to uterine rupture after myomectomy and to refine recommendations for the management of pregnancies in these patients.

RECURRENCE RATES

- A multicentric retrospective cohort study of 512 patients treated with laparoscopic myomectomy postmyomectomy myomas at 5 and 8 years were 53% and 84% respectively; as against this, the rates of reoperation were much lower (7% and 16%, respectively).[11]
- Risk factors for recurrence are multiple myomas at the time of surgery, uterine size ≥13 weeks, and age <36 years.

ALTERNATIVE LAPAROSCOPIC TECHNIQUES

- *Robotics:* Robot-assisted laparoscopic myomectomy has an edge over conventional laparoscopic and open procedures: Laparoscopic suturing may be easier compared to conventional laparoscopy with faster recovery time and lesser blood loss than with open procedures.[12-14] Although it has longer operating times and higher costs, overall outcomes are similar to laparoscopic myomectomy.
- *Single-port laparoscopy:* Single-port laparoscopy, or laparoendoscopic single-site surgery (LESS), refers to a laparoscopic access technique that uses a single incision, usually at the umbilicus.[15] Further studies are needed to evaluate this procedure.
- *Radiofrequency fibroid ablation:* It is an energy-based treatment that reduces fibroid-related symptoms by reducing fibroid volume. It can be done either by hysteroscopic or by laparoscopic approach. After identification of the fibroid by ultrasonography, a conductive needle array punctures the fibroid. A temperature of >100°C is generated which causes coagulative necrosis of the fibroid. Most studies of RFA include small numbers of patients and are limited to fibroids <10 cm and a uterine size ≤16 weeks. It should be used with caution in patients planning pregnancy because of lack of data available as most of the studies evaluating RFA have excluded pregnancy.
- Other infrequently used techniques are laparoscopic uterine artery occlusion and myolysis.

CONCLUSION

Myomectomy involves the surgical removal of leiomyomas from the uterus.

This can be accomplished using an open abdominal, laparoscopic, hysteroscopic, or vaginal approaches.

It is done in patients with symptomatic intramural or subserosal leiomyomas where future childbearing is required.

Imaging methods like pelvic ultrasonography or MRI should be used to confirm the presence of uterine leiomyomas, doing fibroid mapping by assessing their approximate number and location and identifying coincidental lesions like ovarian cysts, which, if present, may impact surgical planning.

The ACOG does not recommend the administration of prophylactic antibiotics for laparoscopic procedures in which the bowel or vagina is not entered.

Laparoscopic myomectomy typically results in lower overall morbidity and a shorter recovery time compared to open myomectomy.

Patients with significant uterine disruption should wait 3–6 months before attempting to conceive.

Alternative laparoscopic techniques include robotics, single-port laparoscopy, radiofrequency fibroid ablation, laparoscopic uterine artery occlusion, and myolysis.

■ REFERENCES

1. Parker WH, Rodi IA. Patient selection for laparoscopic myomectomy. J Am Assoc Gynecol Laparosc. 1994;2:23-6.
2. Dueholm M, Lundorf E, Hansen ES, Ledertoug S, Olesen F. Accuracy of magnetic resonance imaging and transvaginal ultrasonography in the diagnosis, mapping, and measurement of uterine myomas. Am J Obstet Gynecol. 2002;186(3):409-15.
3. ACOG Practice Bulletin No. 195: Prevention of Infection After Gynecologic Procedures. Obstet Gynecol. 2018;131:e172-89.
4. Agarwala N, Liu CY. Safe entry techniques during laparoscopy: left upper quadrant entry using the ninth intercostal space–a review of 918 procedures. J Minim Invasive Gynecol. 2005;12:55-61.
5. Gueye NA, Goodman LR, Falcone T. Versatility of the suprapubic port in robotic assisted laparoscopic myomectomy. Fertil Steril. 2017;108:e1.
6. Sizzi O, Rossetti A, Malzoni M, Minelli L, La Grotta F, Soranna L, et al. Italian multicenter study on complications of laparoscopic myomectomy. J Minim Invasive Gynecol. 2007;14:453-62.
7. Paul GP, Naik SA, Madhu KN, Thomas T. Complications of laparoscopic myomectomy: a single surgeon's series of 1001 cases. Aust N Z J Obstet Gynaecol. 2010;50:385-90.
8. Sinha R, Hegde A, Mahajan C, Dubey N, Sundaram M. Laparoscopic myomectomy: do size, number, and location of the myomas form limiting factors for laparoscopic myomectomy? J Minim Invasive Gynecol 2008;15:292-300.
9. Tsuji S, Takahashi K, Imaoka I, Sugimura K, Miyazaki K, Noda Y. MRI evaluation of the uterine structure after myomectomy. Gynecol Obstet Invest. 2006;61:106-10.
10. Yoo EH, Lee PI, Huh CY, Kim DH, Lee BS, Lee JK, et al. Predictors of leiomyoma recurrence after laparoscopic myomectomy. J Minim Invasive Gynecol. 2007;14:690-7.
11. Advincula AP, Xu X, Goudeau S IV, Ransom SB. Robot-assisted laparoscopic myomectomy versus abdominal myomectomy: a comparison of short-term surgical outcomes and immediate costs. J Minim Invasive Gynecol. 2007;14:698-705.
12. Barakat EE, Bedaiwy MA, Zimberg S, Nutter B, Nosseir M, Falcone T. Robotic-assisted, laparoscopic, and abdominal myomectomy: a comparison of surgical outcomes. Obstet Gynecol. 2011;117:256-66.
13. Ascher-Walsh CJ, Capes TL. Robot-assisted laparoscopic myomectomy is an improvement over laparotomy in women with a limited number of myomas. J Minim Invasive Gynecol. 2010;17:306-10.
14. Kim YW, Park BJ, Ro DY, Kim TE. Single-port laparoscopic myomectomy using a new single-port trans umbilical morcellation system: initial clinical study. J Minim Invasive Gynecol. 2010;17:587-92.
15. Yoshiki N, Okawa T, Kubota T. Single-incision laparoscopic myomectomy with intracorporeal suturing. Fertil Steril. 2011;95:2426-28.

CHAPTER 10

Abdominal Myomectomy

Mitra Saxena

■ INTRODUCTION

"Surgery remains only as safe as those wielding the scalpel."—*Tito Lopes*

Leiomyomas, myomas, or uterine fibroids are the most common benign tumor of females. The treatment options available to manage fibroids are just as myriad as their multiple presentations, ranging from totally asymptomatic to producing numerous symptoms affecting the quality of life. Myomectomy is the surgical removal of fibroid saving the uterus for further reproductive functions or maternal psychological well-being in younger age group patients.

Myomectomy in the current scenario can be carried out by open abdominal method, vaginal route, and laparoscopic route. Depending on the number, size, and location (site: uterus, cervix, and broad ligament), the choice of route of surgery needs to be individualized. The competence and comfort of the operating surgeon play an important role in the final outcome of scheduled surgery.

A review of open myomectomy will be incomplete without mentioning Sir Victor Bonney, who extensively worked on fibroids and carried out 700 surgeries on fibroids in his career and devised multiple techniques and instruments to aid surgical procedure, which was always considered tougher to hysterectomy because of increased expected extra hemorrhage.

■ INDICATIONS

Open abdominal myomectomy is performed for patients who desire future childbearing and in whom symptomatic intramural, transmural or subserosal fibroids, cervical fibroids, or broad ligament fibroids cannot be managed laparoscopically. There will always be a subset of patients where open myomectomy is contraindicated, for example, patient of fibroid with cancer of cervix or uterus or patients where laparotomy is not feasible (medical comorbidities).[1]

■ PRINCIPLES

From the times of Victor Bonney, the following principles have stood test of time, and are applicable, whether myomectomy is performed by open or laparoscopic method:
- Consent
- Technique to reduce intraoperative blood loss
- Planning the incision
- Shelling out the fibroid
- Closing the bed
- Ensuring minimum postoperative adhesions

Informed Consent

Myomectomy is done with the sole purpose of retaining or improving fertility. It is imperative that a detailed explanation of the anticipated benefits and potential complications, including the need for intraoperative hysterectomy, in case of life-threatening hemorrhage,[2] recurrence of fibroids, symptoms, and nonresolution of reproductive issues be discussed with the patient in order to help them make informed decisions. The discussion needs to be documented and informed consent signed in the medical record.

Preoperative Planning

Fibroids come in different sizes, numbers, and sites, posing surgical challenges. With the availability of advanced imaging modalities, that is, 2D, 3D, and MRI, it is now possible to do fibroid mapping preoperatively which helps in counseling and planning surgical incisions over the abdomen/uterus to maximize the results.

Role of GnRH Agonists

Previous authors reported that gonadotropin-releasing hormone (GnRH) agonists reduce uterine size [uterine volume: mean difference (MD)—175 mL; fibroid volume: MD—6 to 155 mL] and there was modest improvement in hemoglobin (MD 0.88 g/dL).[3] This decrease in the size of the fibroid facilitates smaller, transverse abdominal incisions[3] with no significant effect on surgical time or the need for blood transfusion.[3,4]

There are certain negative effects of preoperative GnRH agonists use on the fibroid which are as follows:
- Necrosis of myometrial myoma junction which obscures the tissue planes between the fibroid and normal myometrium making simple enucleation tough and challenging[5]
- Smaller fibroids may shrink and be missed at the time of surgery and later become symptomatic.[5]
- The use of GnRH agonists is thus debatable in the current scenario and in the context of open abdominal myomectomy.

Role of Prophylactic Antibiotics

Prophylactic antibiotics are recommended by American College of Obstetricians and Gynecologists (ACOG) even though the bowel and vagina are not entered. Surgical site infection with open myomectomy is comparable to hysterectomy; additionally, intra-abdominal infection may affect future fertility.[6,7]

Procedure

Anesthesia: Open abdominal myomectomy can be performed under general anesthesia/regional anesthesia.

Use instruments for open myomectomy: Deaver retractors, myomectomy screw, Bonney myomectomy clamp, rubber catheter as tourniquet, vascular clamps, and bulldog are instruments used for open myomectomy.

Skin incision: The skin incision is dependent on the size of uterus/asymmetry due to multiple fibroids/sites of fibroids. A midline vertical incision is used when the uterine size goes beyond 24 weeks, and exteriorizing the uterus is not possible through low transverse abdominal incision (Pfannenstiel/Maylard). A low transverse Pfannenstiel incision suffices for open abdominal myomectomy and to increase the space available, the rectus muscle can be cut (Maylard) **(Fig. 1)**.

Exteriorizing the uterus: Once the uterus is exteriorized from the incision, it puts the uterine vessel on a stretch, which in itself reduces the overall blood supply to the uterus.
- A towel clip/myomectomy screw can be anchored on an identified fibroid to help

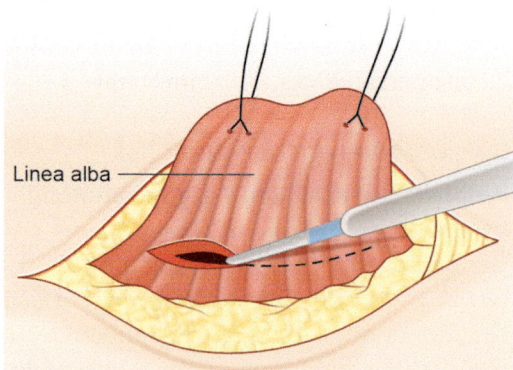

Fig. 1: Pfannenstiel incision. The sheath can be incised transversely and in case more space needed, extended vertically in midline marked as linea alba.

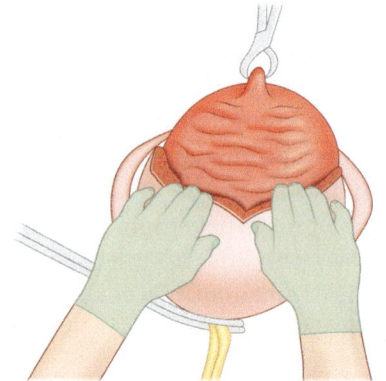

Fig. 2: Use of towel clip to put traction on the fibroid.

in delivering the uterus out of the incision gently **(Figs. 2 and 3)**.
- If one has opened the abdomen transversely and needs the same space to deliver the uterus, the restricting layer, that is, the rectus sheath, can be incised vertically to provide more space, and later at the end of surgery the rectus sheath is closed both vertically and transversally with nonabsorbable/delayed absorbable suture.
- An innovative use of flexible elastic vacuum cup has been used over a fibroid to gently pull out the uterus atraumatically.

Intraoperative Measures to Reduce Blood Loss

- Mechanical
- Vasopressin and other agents

Mechanical

- *Bonney myomectomy clamp* **(Fig. 4)**: A myomectomy clamp devised by Bonney can be placed paracervically as in diagram to cut off blood supply to uterus temporarily. The site of application is the junction between body and cervix.

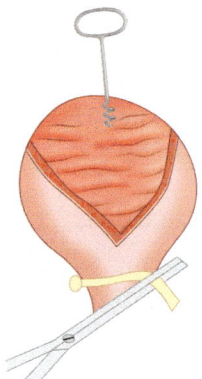

Fig. 3: Use of myomectomy clamp to anchor into fibroid.

- *Uterus and ovarian tourniquet* **(Fig. 5)** Instead of bulky Bonney clamp, temporary rubber tourniquets are placed in the broad ligaments around the ascending branches of uterine vessels on either sides and ring forceps/tourniquets are placed over ovarian vessels through infundibulopelvic ligament.
- *Temporary atraumatic vascular clamp*: Atraumatic vascular bulldog clamps can be put on both internal iliac arteries and vessels medial to the ovaries. All these clamps/tourniquets are removed after the

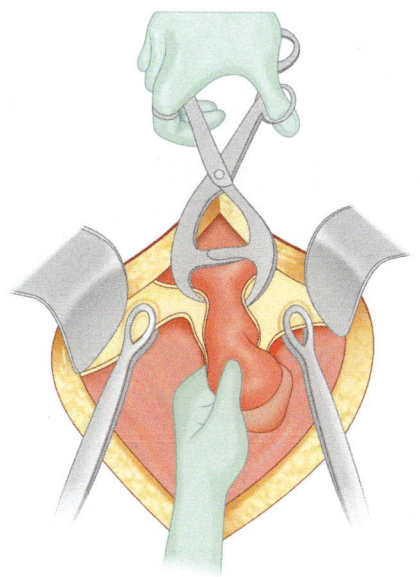

Fig. 4: Application of Bonney clamp.

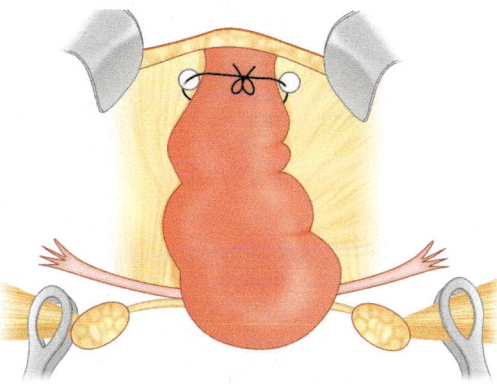

Fig. 5: Tourniquet around uterine vessels.

procedure with no long-term harm to the uterine blood supply.

Use of Vasopressin

Most of the popular agents to decrease blood loss in open or laparoscopic myomectomy is the use of diluted vasopressin (20 units vasopressin in 200 mL normal saline). This is injected after prior information to the anesthetist, subserosally, taking full precaution to avoid accidental injection in a vessel. In case the procedure is prolonged, it can be reinjected after 30 minutes. It is advisable to be swift and cautious to work efficiently.

Incision Over Uterus

After exteriorization of the uterus, all fibroids are palpated and the incision on the uterus is planned.

- For a strong subsequent scar, a lower incision over the anterior aspect of the uterus is preferred.
- It is advisable to remove maximum fibroids from a single midline incision when possible.
- Incision over the anterior aspect of the uterus has lower adhesions as compared to the posterior wall.
- Extension of incision into cornua and uterine vessels has to be avoided, especially when fibroids are multiple and distort the normal vascular architecture.
- If there are fibroids on the anterior and posterior walls, then separate incisions can be made to avoid going through the endometrial cavity.
- In case the endometrial cavity gets opened inadvertently. Repair of the myoma bed is done meticulously. The integrity of endometrial cavity is ensured by placing a pediatric Foley's catheter with inflated bulb.[8-12]

Single/Multiple Incision

Economy of incision over the uterus has to be weighed against burrowing through a single incision to extract distant myomas which can cause tunneling defects in the myometrium which will be difficult to close and interfere with hemostasis. Incision over the uterus can be made with a needle-tip

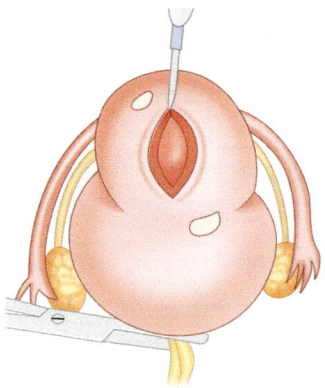

Fig. 6: Incision up to pseudocapsule with monopolar tip.

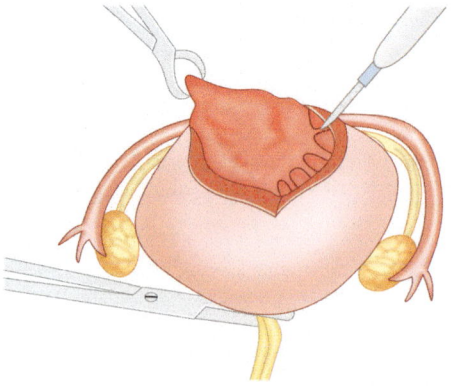

Fig. 7: Base of fibroid vessels coagulated before removing it completely.

monopolar electrosurgical instrument or scalpel **(Fig. 6)**. The incision should extend below the pseudocapsule to work in the avascular surgical plane. Once within the correct avascular surgical plane, the fibroid bulges and becomes visible.

Removal or Shelling of the Myomas

A myomectomy clamp or a towel clip can be anchored to the fibroid and continuous upward traction is applied **(Figs. 2 and 3)**. Pseudocapsule is bluntly or sharply dissected from the fibroid till it is shelled out completely. Electrosurgical tip can be used to separate and coagulate bed from the fibroid **(Fig. 7)**. Fibroid has a rich vascular supply and excessive bleeding has to be taken care of by previously mentioned procedures.

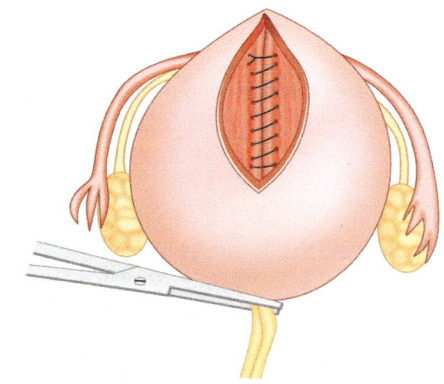

Fig. 8: Layered closure; simple running continuous in base.

Closure of the Bed

Myometrial defect is closed by using 0 vicryl suture **(Fig. 8)**. If defect is >2 cm deep, layered closure is recommended to achieve adequate tissue apposition and complete hemostasis. The serosa is closed by baseball stitch (inside out) with finer suture 2-0 vicryl/monocryl to decrease exposure of suture/subsequent adhesion formation **(Fig. 9)**.

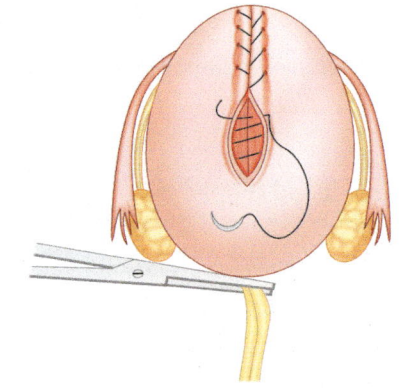

Fig. 9: Serosa, closed by baseball suture (inside out).

Adhesion prevention:
- Complete hemostasis
- Layered closure
- Perfect apposition
- Minimal incisions
- Use of Interceed

Abdominal closure: Routine closure of all layers is recommended. The most important is closure of the fascial sheath including extensions, if any.

Role of Postoperative Pain Management and Thromboprophylaxis

In abdominal open myomectomy, postoperative pain needs to be managed adequately with analgesics (PCM) and opioid alkaloids subject to availability.

Cervical fibroid is rare, 0.6%. It can cause reproductive failures by causing anatomic endocervical blockages, recurrent pregnancy losses, and obstructed labor. MRI needs to be done preoperatively to plan the myomectomy. Bilateral ligation of the uterine artery at the origin or anterior division of Internal Iliac Artery ligation can be done to decrease intraoperative hemorrhage. The relationship of ureters has to be kept in mind while dissecting, shelling out fibroid, and closing the bed. It is always recommended to stay within the pseudocapsule, and put traction, and do sharp dissection with the tip of instrument that is visible.

Broad ligament fibroids: The principles for open myomectomy remain the same. In true broad ligament fibroids, the uterine vessels are medial and ureters are lateral to the fibroids.

■ COMPLICATIONS

Open myomectomy is a major surgery and riddled with hemorrhage infection, fever adhesion, hysterectomy, paralytic ileus, and visceral injury.

Hemorrhage: The amount of blood loss is variable from 200 to 800 mL,[13,14] and requirement of blood transfusion varies from 2 to 28%.[13-16] Big size and entering into uterine cavity are associated with more blood loss.[17] Less than 4% are converted to hysterectomy due to inoperability or hemorrhage.[18,19]

Fever and Infection

Fever in the first 24–48 hours is attributed to systemic inflammatory response syndrome (SIRS)[18,19] so unless there are localizing signs, this is to be managed symptomatically. A hematoma is to be avoided by meticulous layered closure.

Unplanned hysterectomy: Limited data are available on conversion to hysterectomy with incidence reported as low as <1%[20] to 3.2%.[21]

Adhesions: Myomectomies are notorious for postoperative adhesions, especially due to incisions on the posterior aspect and due to sutures.

Follow-up and Counseling

Patients should be mobile in the immediate postoperative period with early resumption of oral intake for enhanced recovery after surgery (ERAS). The patient is fit for normal activities within a fortnight and can resume sexual activity in 6 weeks; however, planning the next pregnancy has to be delayed for at least 3–6 months.[22]

Rupture of Myomectomy Scar

The risk of rupture of a myomectomy scar is increased when there is extensive surgery and when complicated with the opening of the endometrial cavity. The decision for elective cesarean section needs to be individualized and the patient managed as a high risk.

CONCLUSION

Open myomectomy is a very rewarding surgery for complicated, multiple fibroids distorting the shape and size of the uterus. Although laparoscopic removal is much in demand and being done very frequently, the expertise of all endoscopic surgeons is not at par. Upgradation of multiple energy sources and suture materials are means to flatten the learning curve; however, good surgical principles for myomectomy are to be followed in the best of hands endoscopically or by open method.

REFERENCES

1. Parker WH, Sharp HT, Chakrabarti A. Uterine fibroids (leiomyomas): Prolapsed fibroids. UpToDate. 2023;1:16.
2. Management of Symptomatic Uterine Leiomyomas: ACOG Practice Bulletin, Number 228. Obstet Gynecol. 2021;137(6).
3. Lethaby A, Puscasiu L, Vollenhoven B. Preoperative medical therapy before surgery for uterine fibroids. Cochrane Database Syst Rev. 2017;11(11):CD000547.
4. Deligdisch L, Hirschmann S, Altchek A. Pathologic changes in gonadotropin-releasing hormone agonist analogue treated uterine leiomyomata. Fertil Steril. 1997;67(5):837-41.
5. ACOG Practice Bulletin No. 195: Prevention of Infection After Gynecologic Procedures. Obstet Gynecol. 2018;131(6):e172-89.
6. Mukhopadhaya N, De Silva C, Manyonda IT. Conventional myomectomy. Best Pract Res Clin Obstet Gynaecol. 2008;22(4):677-705.
7. Discepola F, Valenti DA, Reinhold C, Tulandi T. Analysis of arterial blood vessels surrounding the myoma: Relevance to myomectomy. Obstet Gynecol. 2007;110(6):1301-3.
8. Tulandi T, Murray C, Guralnick M. Adhesion formation and reproductive outcome after myomectomy and second-look laparoscopy. Obstet Gynecol. 1993;82(2):213-5.
9. Guarnaccia MM, Rein MS. Traditional surgical approaches to uterine fibroids: Abdominal myomectomy and hysterectomy. Clin Obstet Gynecol. 2001;44(2):385-400.
10. West S, Ruiz R, Parker WH. Abdominal myomectomy in women with very large uterine size. Fertil Steril. 2006;85(1):36-9.
11. Walocha JA, Litwin JA, Miodoński AJ. Vascular system of intramural leiomyomata revealed by corrosion casting and scanning electron microscopy. Hum Reprod. 2003; 18(5):1088-93.
12. Bhandari S, Ganguly I, Agarwal P, Singh A, Gupta N. Effect of myomectomy on endometrial cavity: A prospective study of 51 cases. J Hum Reprod Sci. 2016;9(2):107-11.
13. Sawin SW, Pilevsky ND, Berlin JA, Barnhart KT. Comparability of perioperative morbidity between abdominal myomectomy and hysterectomy for women with uterine leiomyomas. Am J Obstet Gynecol. 2000; 183(6):1448-55.
14. Iverson RE Jr, Chelmow D, Strohbehn K, Waldman L, Evantash EG. Relative morbidity of abdominal hysterectomy and myomectomy for management of uterine leiomyomas. Obstet Gynecol. 1996;88(3):415-9.
15. Kim T, Purdy MP, Kendall-Rauchfuss L, Habermann EB, Bews KA, Glasgow AE, et al. Myomectomy associated blood transfusion risk and morbidity after surgery. Fertil Steril. 2020;114(1):175-84.
16. LaMorte AI, Lalwani S, Diamond MP. Morbidity associated with abdominal myomectomy. Obstet Gynecol. 1993;82(6): 897-900.
17. Schüring AN, Garcia-Rocha GJ, Schlösser HW, Greb RR, Kiesel L, Schippert C. Perioperative complications in conventional and microsurgical abdominal myomectomy. Arch Gynecol Obstet. 2011;284(1):137-44.
18. Hartmann KE, Fonnesbeck C, Surawicz T, Krishnaswami S, Andrews JC, Wilson JE, et al. Management of Uterine Fibroids. Rockville (MD): Agency for Healthcare Research and Quality (US); 2017.

19. Olufowobi O, Sharif K, Papaionnou S, Neelakantan D, Mohammed H, Afnan M. Are the anticipated benefits of myomectomy achieved in women of reproductive age? A 5-year review of the results at a UK tertiary hospital. J Obstet Gynaecol. 2004;24(4):434-40.
20. Mirowska-Allen KL, Kong KK, Ang WC. Unplanned hysterectomy following myomectomy at a tertiary institution: A case series and review of the literature. J Endometriosis Pelvic Pain Disord. 2018;10(3):151-7.
21. Coyne K, Purdy MP, Bews KA, Habermann EB, Khan Z. Risk of hysterectomy at the time of myomectomy: An underestimated surgical risk. Fertil Steril. 2024;121(1):107-16.
22. Tsuji S, Takahashi K, Imaoka I, Sugimura K, Miyazaki K, Noda Y. MRI evaluation of the uterine structure after myomectomy. Gynecol Obstet Invest. 2006;61(2):106-10.

CHAPTER 11

Hysteroscopic Myomectomy

Kavita Agarwal

INTRODUCTION

Uterine myomas are benign tumors formed of smooth muscle cells with variable amount of connective tissue. They constitute 20% of all benign tumors. Most of the symptoms are produced by submucous myomas and hence are considered to be most troublesome. They can result in abnormal uterine bleeding, pelvic pain, dysmenorrhea, infertility, and recurrent miscarriage. The standard approach for resection of symptomatic submucous myomas is by hysteroscopy through uterine cervix.

PREOPERATIVE EVALUATION OF MYOMAS

The evaluation of submucous myomas includes transvaginal ultrasound (TVS), saline infusion sonography (SIS), and hysteroscopy. TVS can easily determine the size of submucous myoma and its location and degree of intramural extension. Magnetic resonance imaging (MRI) is more sensitive than TVS for topographic study of fibroids and can also distinguish between fibroids and adenomyosis. SIS can precisely diagnose myoma location, its penetration into myometrium, and distance of free myometrium between the myoma and serosa. Although hysteroscopy does not precisely evaluate intramyometrial extension and distance between myoma and serosa, which can be determined by TVS and SIS, hysteroscopy provides definitive diagnosis of submucous myoma. Hysteroscopy can distinguish between submucous myoma and endometrial polyp and confirm the number of submucous myomas and their precise location. Hysteroscopy is considered to be the method of choice for assessing the feasibility of hysteroscopic resection.

Lasmar et al.[1] in 2005 proposed a STEP-W classification including the parameters: Size of myoma, topography, extension of base of nodule with respect to uterine wall, penetration into myometrium and wall from which myoma arises. Score ranging from 0 to 2 is given for each parameter and then patients are allocated into one of the three groups **(Table 1)**. This scoring system correlates with completeness of myomectomy, fluid deficit, and time spent in surgery.

ANESTHESIA

Regional anesthesia is preferred to general anesthesia to monitor the clinical manifestations of fluid intoxication. The chief manifestations are nausea, vomiting, headache, disorientation, etc.

SURGICAL TECHNIQUE OF HYSTEROSCOPIC MYOMECTOMY

Surgery should be done in the proliferative phase of menstrual cycle as the endometrium is thin with less vascularity.

TABLE 1: STEP-W classification.[1]					
	Size	Penetration	Base	Topography	Lateral wall
0	≤2 cm	0	≤1/3	Lower	
1	>2–5 cm	≤50%	>1/3 to 2/3	Middle	+1
2	>5 cm	>50%	>2/3	Upper	
Score		+	+	+	
Score	Group	Suggested treatment			
0–4	I	Low complexity hysteroscopic myomectomy			
5–6	II	Complex hysteroscopic myomectomy, consider preparing with GnRH analog and/or two-step surgery			
7–9	III	Recommend an alternative nonhysteroscopic technique			

(GnRH: gonadotropin-releasing hormone)

Slicing Technique

Monopolar uses glycine as a distension medium. Bipolar is safer and uses saline solution as a distension medium. The vessels over the surface of the myoma are to be coagulated before beginning the resection procedure. It reduces the amount of bleeding and fluid absorption during the procedure. The loop electrode is attached to the resectoscope and slicing is started from beyond the myoma. The loop should always be moved forward from behind the myoma in a forward direction, i.e., from the fundus to the internal os. The electrode should be kept in view during the entire procedure. Slicing is done from the top of the myoma toward its base and is done till the fasciculate structure of myometrium is visualized. This is identified by the pinkest color and soft consistency and it bleeds easily. The damage to the adjacent endometrium should be avoided during resection and pure cutting current should be set. The inflow and outflow of distension medium should be monitored. The fragments need to be intermittently removed from the uterine cavity for better vision. At the completion of the procedure, inspect the cavity and bleeders, if any, need to be coagulated.

Challenging Myomas

Myomas which are large in size, located at the fundus, and penetrating deep into myometrium are challenging.

Preoperative Hormonal Treatment

Preoperative treatment with gonadotropin-releasing hormone (GnRH) analogs for 2–3 months offers advantages by shrinking myoma by 30–50%, reducing fibroid vascularity and reducing the duration of surgery. However, it increases the cost of the treatment and also side effects related to estrogen withdrawal.

Bringing Intramural Component into the Cavity

- Wait for a few seconds to allow uterine contractions to cause the intramural portion of the myoma to protrude into the uterine cavity.
- Intermittent release of intrauterine pressure helps myoma protrude into the uterine cavity.

- Use of intravenous oxytocin to stimulate uterine contractions for expulsion of intramural portion of the myoma. Murakami et al.[2] used prostaglandin F2 (PGF2) alpha intra-abdominal injection under laparoscopic guidance and Indman[3] used intracervical carboprost to facilitate hysteroscopic resection of submucous fibroids.
- *Complete excision in two-step procedure:* The first step is to resect the intracavitary portion of the myoma. The second surgical step for complete excision is scheduled 1 month later after the first menstruation and after confirming migration of the residual intramural component by office hysteroscopy.

Alternative Techniques

- *Vaporization:* The Versapoint system vaporizes the myoma using a 200W bipolar current. It uses saline for distension medium and can be used only for type 0 and type 1 myomas with size <2 cm. There is a risk of perforation as prolonged pressure in one spot. Also, no tissue is available for histopathology.
- *Ablation of myoma:* Small, <2 cm myomas can be ablated using neodymium-doped yttrium–aluminum–garnet (Nd-YAG) laser. The major disadvantage is lack of tissue sample for pathology.
- *Intrauterine morcellator:* The hysteroscopic morcellator does mechanical cutting by the rotation of the internal tube of morcellator. Hence, it reduces the tumor into small pieces. At the same time, the cut pieces are evacuated out of the uterine cavity by aspiration. It uses saline solution as a distension medium. This is a safe and effective procedure. Also, it eliminates the need to remove the fragments with the hysteroscope.

POSTOPERATIVE CARE

Monitoring of vitals should be done in the immediate postoperative period. Analgesics like nonsteroidal anti-inflammatory drugs (NSAIDs) should be prescribed. The patient can be discharged after 4 hours with recommended rest for 24–48 hours.

COMPLICATIONS OF HYSTEROSCOPIC MYOMECTOMY

The most common complications are related to distension media and uterine perforation. The other complications include bleeding, air embolism, infection, and postoperative adhesions.

Complications due to distension medium include excessive intravasation and hyponatremia. This can be avoided by strict monitoring of inflow and outflow of fluid during the procedure. Hyponatremia can be avoided by using normal saline as a distension medium with bipolar energy.[4]

Uterine perforation may occur during dilatation of cervix, insertion of hysteroscope, and during resection of the intramural part of myoma. As soon as perforation is detected, the procedure should be immediately stopped. Perforation with an activated electrode necessitates laparoscopy/laparotomy to exclude bowel injury.

Bleeding after hysteroscopic myomectomy can be controlled by insertion of Foley's catheter with 30cc saline instillation. The balloon can be maintained for 24 hours. Thereafter, it can be gradually deflated and Foley's catheter removed.

Postoperative uterine adhesions are especially seen in fibroids located on opposite endometrial surfaces, especially anterior and posterior sides. They can be prevented by reducing the use of electrosurgery and by administration of estrogens for endometrial regeneration.

◼ CONCLUSION

Hysteroscopic myomectomy in the present era is a standard management of submucous myomas. The right selection of cases by proper preoperative evaluation to determine the feasibility of hysteroscopic resection is the key to success of the procedure. Also, improved skill, experience, inflow, outflow of fluid monitoring, and proper technique are crucial to avoid complications of the procedure.

◼ REFERENCES

1. Lasmar RB, Barrozo PR, Dias R, Oliveira MA. Submucous fibroids: a new presurgical classification to evaluate the viability of hysteroscopic surgical treatment—preliminary report. J Minim Invasive Gynecol. 2005;12:308-11.
2. Murakami T, Tachiban M, Hoshiai T, Osawa Y, Terada Y, Okamura K. Successful strategy for the hysteroscopic myomectomy of a submucous fibroid arising from the uterine fundus. Fertile Steril. 2006;86:1513.
3. Indman PD. Use of carboprost to facilitate hysteroscopic resection of submucous fibroids. J Am Assoc. Gynecol Laparosc. 2004; 11:68-72.
4. Darwish AM, Hassan ZZ, Attia AM, Abdelraheem SS, Ahmed YM. Biological effects of distension media in bipolar versus monopolar resectoscopic myomectomy: a randomized trial. J Obstet Gynaecol Res. 2010;36:810-7.

Intrauterine System in Fibroids: An Effective Treatment Option

Parag Biniwale, Amrita Saha

■ INTRODUCTION

Fibroids are the predominant neoplasms found within the pelvic region of women.[1] Benign tumors, known as fibroids, appear in around 30–50% of women above the age of 35 years, with a higher prevalence seen among black women.[2] Fibroids can manifest in different forms, including submucosal fibroids, which grow into the uterine cavity, and pedunculated fibroids, which are attached to the uterus by a stalk-like structure. Although the exact cause of fibroids remains unclear, they are essentially tumors that originate from the smooth muscle of the uterus, and their growth is influenced by estrogen and progesterone, which are ovarian steroids. Estrogen and estradiol prompt the production of estrogen receptor (ER) alpha, which in turn enhances the expression of progesterone receptor (PR). The presence of PR is essential for fibroids to respond to progesterone. In the absence of progesterone and PR, the presence of estrogen and ER alpha alone is insufficient for the growth of fibroids.[3]

In many women, fibroids are asymptomatic, and they do not require any treatment. The bleeding that occurs due to the presence of fibroids seems to be linked to changes in the endometrial tissue at a histological and hormonal level. These changes result in the destabilization of the endometrial vascular system, potentially leading to irregular bleeding.[4] Pelvic pressure or pain, obstructive symptoms, infertility, urinary disorders, and recurrent pregnancy loss are other symptoms that negatively impact the quality of health of females.

Surgery is considered the primary approach in treating symptomatic fibroids. However, pharmacological and updated minimally invasive techniques are showing promising results. One such technique is the levonorgestrel-releasing intrauterine system (LNG IUS), which has been available in the market since 1990. It is a small T-shaped device that is inserted into the uterus to release a controlled amount of levonorgestrel (52 mg), a synthetic progesterone hormone, at a rate of 20 µg/day for a long period (up to 5 years). LNG IUS is highly effective as a contraceptive device, with less than 1% failure rate, and is also approved for the treatment of heavy menstrual bleeding (HMB), endometrial hyperplasia, and as an adjuvant therapy for endometriosis.

■ MECHANISM OF ACTION

The LNG IUS works through a combination of local and systemic effects. Locally, levonorgestrel applied by the LNG IUS significantly impacts the functional endometrium by effectively suppressing its activity while also promoting the thickening of cervical mucus.[5] Systemically, the LNG IUS suppresses the production of follicle-stimulating hormone (FSH) and luteinizing hormone (LH), which helps reduce the size of fibroids and control symptoms associated with fibroids. Additionally, LNG IUS is responsible for increasing uterine artery resistance index (RI) and reducing the size of uterine volume.[6] This contributes to the reduction in bleeding and pain associated with fibroids. However, it does not have any impact on the size of the fibroids themselves.

■ EFFECT ON FIBROIDS

Although the LNG IUS does not provide a direct cure for fibroids, it has been shown to alleviate many symptoms associated with this benign tumor. The continuous release of levonorgestrel into the uterus suppresses the growth of fibroids by downregulating the ERs in the endometrium. This leads to a reduction in fibroid-related bleeding, pain, and discomfort. Starczewski et al. highlighted that the LNG IUS offers additional advantages beyond contraception, such as diminishing the amount of menstrual bleeding and decreasing the size of the uterus.[7] Another research study supporting the favorable impact of LNG IUS on HMB demonstrated that women using LNG showed an increase in levels of hemoglobin, hematocrit, and ferritin.[8] Additionally, after a follow-up period of 3 years, Magalhães J et al. observed that women using LNG IUS experienced a considerable decrease in uterine volume, with a mean reduction from 156.6 to 90 cm^3. However, the volume of fibroids remained the same and unaffected.[9]

On the contrary, Socolov et al. reported that while the LNG IUS is effective in managing HMB associated with the presence of fibroids, it does not significantly impact the size of the tumors.[10] Additionally, a recent systematic review highlighted LNG IUS as a potential recommended treatment option specifically for menorrhagia caused by uterine fibroids.[10]

■ INDICATIONS AND CONTRAINDICATIONS

The LNG IUS presents a promising treatment option for certain symptoms associated with uterine fibroids. Indications for its use include the management of HMB and other symptoms like pelvic pain and discomfort. However, it is essential to recognize its limitations and contraindications.

The LNG IUS should not be prescribed in certain types of fibroids:
- *Submucosal fibroids:* These fibroids protrude into the uterine cavity and can cause significant symptoms such as HMB. While LNG IUS can help manage the bleeding, it may not effectively treat the underlying cause. Surgical interventions like hysteroscopic resection or myomectomy are often more appropriate for this type of fibroid.
- *Pedunculated fibroids:* These fibroids are attached to the uterus by a stalk or stem, and they can be located inside or outside the uterus. LNG IUS may not be effective in treating these fibroids, as the levonorgestrel released by the device primarily acts within the uterus. Surgical removal of pedunculated fibroids is typically the recommended treatment approach.

It is crucial for healthcare providers to carefully evaluate the type and location of fibroids before prescribing LNG IUS. A thorough assessment can help determine the most appropriate treatment option for individual patients.

PATIENT COUNSELING AND FOLLOW-UP

Before recommending LNG IUS for the treatment of fibroids, thorough counseling is essential. Patients should be informed about the procedure for device insertion, potential side effects such as irregular bleeding during the initial months followed by amenorrhea in some women, and the importance of regular follow-up visits. It is important to convey that it may take several months for the full effect of the device to be noticeable and that alternative treatment options, including surgery, may be necessary in some cases. Addressing any concerns or questions the patient may have during the counseling session is crucial.

After LNG IUS insertion, regular follow-up visits are necessary to monitor the patient's response and ensure optimal treatment outcomes. The first follow-up visit should be scheduled around 4-6 weeks after insertion to assess side effects, review symptom improvement, and check for proper device placement. Subsequent visits can be scheduled every 3-6 months or as indicated by the patient's symptoms. It is crucial to assess the patient's overall satisfaction, monitor the reduction in fibroid size if applicable, and address any concerns or side effects that may arise.

DISCUSSION ON STUDIES AND POTENTIAL RISKS

A study has highlighted the efficacy of LNG IUS in managing symptoms associated with fibroids, particularly in reducing menstrual bleeding and decreasing uterine volume.[8] However, it is important to note that LNG IUS may not have a significant impact on the size of the fibroids themselves, as mentioned by Socolov et al.[10]

While LNG IUS presents benefits in symptom management, it is important to discuss potential risks or downsides with patients. These may include irregular bleeding during the initial months, amenorrhea, potential expulsion of the device, and the need for surgical intervention in certain cases where LNG IUS may not be effective.

PATIENT EDUCATION ON ALTERNATIVE TREATMENT OPTIONS

In addition to discussing LNG IUS as a treatment option, it is crucial to provide patients with information on alternative treatment options for fibroids. This includes surgical interventions such as myomectomy or hysterectomy, minimally invasive procedures such as uterine artery embolization, and nonsurgical options such as hormonal therapy or watchful waiting. Each option comes with its own benefits and risks, and patients should be empowered to make informed decisions about their treatment based on their individual circumstances and preferences.

CONCLUSION

The LNG IUS offers a valuable treatment option for women with symptomatic fibroids, particularly those seeking contraception. While LNG IUS effectively suppresses fibroid growth and alleviates associated symptoms, such as HMB, it is important to acknowledge its limitations, including its potential lack of impact on fibroid size. Patient counseling and regular follow-up visits are essential for optimizing treatment outcomes. Despite these considerations, LNG IUS remains a valuable tool in managing HMB associated with fibroids, offering a less invasive alternative to surgical procedures.

REFERENCES

1. Buttram VC. Uterine leiomyomata—aetiology, symptomatology and management. Prog Clin Biol Res. 1986;225:275-96.
2. Baird DD, Dunson DB, Hill MC, Cousins D, Schectman JM. High cumulative incidence of uterine leiomyoma in black and white women: ultrasound evidence. Am J Obstet Gynecol. 2003;188(1):100-7.
3. Bulun SE. Uterine fibroids. N Engl J Med. 2013;369:1344-55.
4. Maia H, Pimentel K, Casoy J, Correia T, Antonio R Freitas L, Zausner B, et al. Aromatase expression in the eutopic endometrium of myomatous uteri: the influence of the menstrual cycle and oral contraceptive use. Gynecol Endocrinol. 2007;23(6):320-4.
5. Bayer LL, Hillard PJA. Use of levonorgestrel intrauterine system for medical indications in adolescents. J Adolesc Heal. 2013;52(4 Suppl):S54-8.
6. Haberal A, Kayikcioglu F, Gunes M, Kaplan M, Ozdegirmenci O. The effect of the levonorgestrel intrauterine system on uterine artery blood flow 1 year after insertion. Ultrasound Obstet Gynecol. 2006;27(3):316-9.
7. Starczewski A, Iwanicki M. Intrauterine therapy with levonorgestrel releasing IUD of women with hypermenorrhea secondary to uterine fibroids. Ginekol Pol. 2000;71(9):1221-5.
8. Zapata LB, Whiteman MK, Tepper NK, Jamieson DJ, Marchbanks PA, Curtis KM. Intrauterine device use among women with uterine fibroids: a systematic review. Contraception. 2010;82(1):41-55.
9. Magalhães J, Aldrighi JM, de Lima GR. Uterine volume and menstrual patterns in users of the levonorgestrel-releasing intrauterine system with idiopathic menorrhagia or menorrhagia due to leiomyomas. Contraception. 2007;75(3):193-8.
10. Socolov D, Blidaru I, Tamba B, Miron N, Boiculese L, Socolov R. Levonorgestrel releasing intrauterine system for the treatment of menorrhagia and/or frequent irregular uterine bleeding associated with uterine leiomyoma. Eur J Contracept Reprod Heal Care. 2011;16(6):480-7.

CHAPTER 13

Sexual and Psychosexual Dysfunction

Monisha Singh, Neharika Malhotra

INTRODUCTION

Symptomatic uterine fibroids greatly affect the daily living and quality of life of women who have them. While the physical outcomes of uterine fibroids have been well documented, little investment has been made into research around their impact on a woman's emotional, mental, and psychological well-being.

Because uterine fibroids impact a wide cross-section of the female population, we must understand implications of the physical outcomes of symptomatic uterine fibroids. Negative outcomes include, but are not limited to, concerns around self-image, inadequacy, helplessness, loss of control, and severe impact on the self-esteem of a woman. In turn, these concerns and emotions may have an effect on the sexual function and vitality of a woman's sexual health. For example, the physical appearance of having uterine fibroids can sometimes be confused with appearing to be pregnant or overweight leading to a woman's decreased sense of comfort in her own skin.

To better serve and support individuals living with symptomatic uterine fibroids, providers, physicians, community advocates, and activists need to understand the overreaching impact that uterine fibroids have on the women who have to confront their existence every day. Despite the high prevalence of uterine fibroids, the psychosocial impact of fibroids has not been evaluated across different quality of life indicators and compared with other chronic conditions. Sexual dysfunction in premenopausal women is quite common affecting around one-third of women, and presence of fibroids adds to such dysfunction.

EFFECT OF FIBROIDS ON QUALITY OF LIFE

- Heavy menstrual bleeding (HMB) alongside dyspareunia could hamper sexual arousal, which indirectly reduced the frequency of intercourse, resulting in subfertility.
- Sometimes, presence of fibroids has a significant association with deep dyspareunia and impaired sexual satisfaction. Fundal fibroids were highly associated with dyspareunia amongst all locations.
- Treatment of fibroids, like myomectomy, may relieve pelvic pain during intercourse, thereby improving sexual function in these women. The pudendal nerve injury posthysterectomy can contribute to sexual impairment. In conclusion, sexual dysfunction in an infertile couple is a complex issue and, along with possible treatment of fibroids, it might be necessary to also address other medical or psychosocial problems.[1]

ANATOMY AND PHYSIOLOGICAL FUNCTION OF FEMALE SEXUAL FUNCTION

The pelvic autonomic nerves supply the blood vessels of the vaginal wall, which originate mostly from the inferior hypogastric plexus (IHP). The IHP is essential for lubrication and sensation of the internal genitalia.

The sensation of the external genitalia is linked to the pudendal nerve; this somatosensory nerve supplies the labia and clitoris and reaches the external genitalia through a canal within the pelvic floor **(Fig. 1)**.

HOW FIBROIDS CAUSE PAIN DURING SEX

Fibroids cause symptom and dyspareunia based on their location. Sexual dysfunction can occur from pelvic pain, dyspareunia, and HMB, which interferes with sexual arousal.

- *Cervical fibroids:* One near cervix or near os can cause pain during penetration and the resulting friction can also be very uncomfortable and can cause spotting.
- Fibroids that are growing on the upper portion of the uterus can cause painful pressure during sex accompanied by cramping or shooting stomach pains. Women have even reported having stomach pains for hours after intercourse.
- The submucosal fibroid may definitely present as HMB which may indirectly cause weakness and anemia. The subserosal kind, especially the large ones, may push against pelvic nerves to cause pelvic pain and pressure-related symptoms, like polyuria and nocturia **(Fig. 2)**.
- Intramural fibroids can cause either bleeding or pain or both depending on which way they grow, i.e., inwardly or outwardly.
- Individuals with symptomatic fibroids are often reluctant to discuss this issue as it involves having to confront feelings of inadequacy and rejection.[2]

Many studies have suggested a positive correlation of sexual dysfunction post hysterectomy with disruption of the autonomic nerve supply. The disruption of the IHP can lead to altered lubrication and differed sensation of the internal genital organs. In addition, some research has suggested that the removal of the cervix can eliminate internal orgasm.

For instance, external orgasm is reliant on the pudendal nerve which supplies sensation to the labia and clitoris. Both can be affected by surgical intervention harming the sexual function.[3]

CAUSE OF PSYCHOSEXUAL DYSFUNCTION

The psychological impact of fibroid on a woman is a significant one where the woman undergoes anxiety to mild depression. Such cases should not be taken lightly and all queries regarding sex must be answered by the gynecologist.

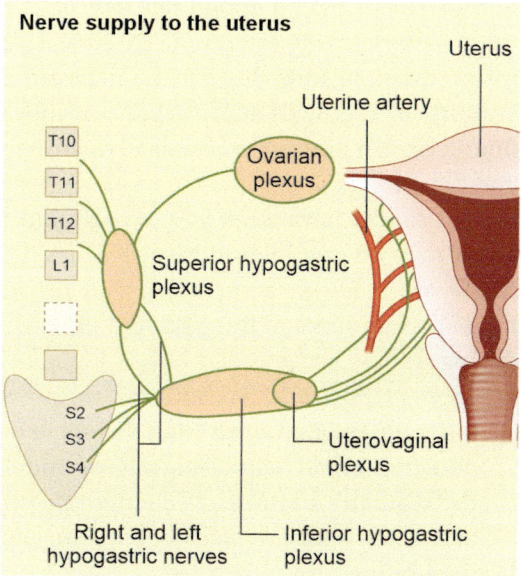

Fig. 1: Innervation of uterus and its adnexa.

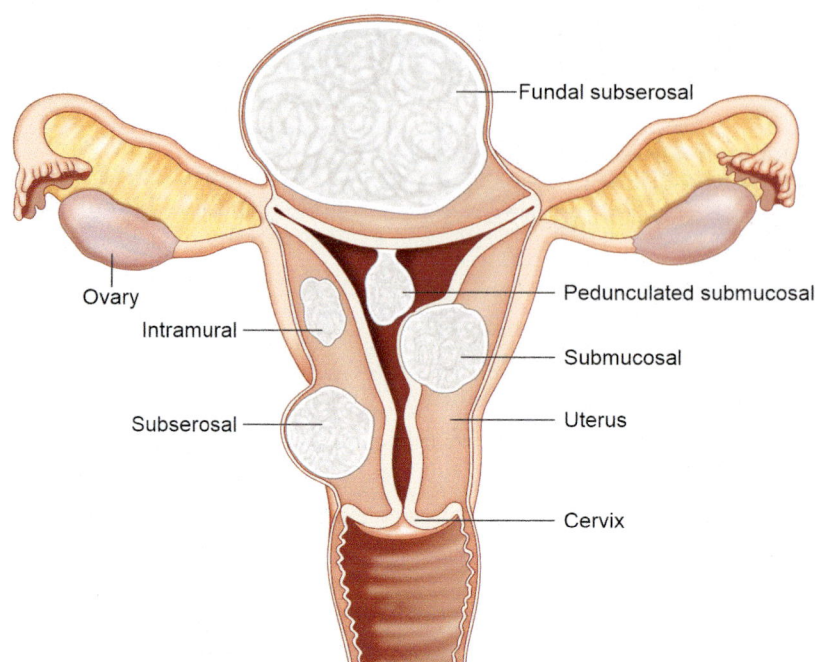

Fig. 2: Various locations of fibroid in uterus.
Courtesy: Mayo Foundation for Medical Education and Research.

- Fibroids can cause agony to such an extent that a woman will avert any sexual position or abstain from sex altogether.
- Sometimes, fibroids cause bleeding after sex which can cause embarrassment and result in the woman avoiding intimacy.
- A woman can feel irritable, worn out, uncomfortable, and not feel desirable or self-confident in her ability to please her sexual partner.
- Hormone imbalances that alter a woman's libido can be caused by fibroids. This can place a significant tension in a relation.
- Fibroids that lead to heavy bleeding can result in anemia which can cause fatigue, lethargy, severe headaches, etc. Women with chronic anemia will cause a diminished lifestyle to the point that having sex with fibroids becomes a difficult task.

■ MANAGEMENT

The psychological distress secondary to fibroids does not end upon their removal, as the risk of regrowth is around 15–30%. As a result, multiple surgeries may be necessary. Waiting for regrowth after surgery, or more fibroid growth presurgery, can lead to anxiety and dread.

It is safe to have sex if you have fibroids, but it may be painful and less pleasurable. There are a few strategies you can try to help alleviate some of the pain and pressure during sex.[4]

- *Change position:* Sometimes trying a different position or shifting the angle of penetration can help. Using pillows under the woman's buttocks to change the tilt of her pelvis may reduce or eliminate any discomfort.

- Increasing the length of foreplay may help increase pleasure and lessen discomfort.
- Pleasure each other in different ways and avoid penetration.

CONCLUSION

Leiomyomas are quite prevalent in reproductive and perimenopausal age-group. Many such space-occupying lesions in itself can cause sexual dysfunction owing to pelvic pain, dyspareunia and HMB. Their management including medical and surgical may sometimes heal such symptoms, although sometimes these treatment in itself may rarely cause further psychological or psychosexual health issues. A fine discussion with a gynecologist is necessary to elaborate a plan for treatment of such a condition, and while healing is essential, one should also focus on a woman's sexual needs and comfort too.

REFERENCES

1. Go VAA, Thomas MC, Singh B, Prenatt S, Sims H, Blanck JF, et al. A systematic review of the psychosocial impact of fibroids before and after treatment. Am J Obstet Gynecol. 2020;223(5):674-708.e8.
2. Louie AR, Armstrong JA, Findeiss LK, Goodwin SC. Comparison of sexual dysfunction using the female sexual function index following surgical treatments for uterine fibroids. Case Rep Obstet Gynecol. 2012;2012:368136.
3. Don EE, Mijatovic V, Huirne JAF. Infertility in patients with uterine fibroids: a debate about the hypothetical mechanisms. Hum Reprod. 2023;38(11):2045-54.
4. Chang JH, Shin DW, Jeon MJ, Hong H, Kim SM, An A, et al. Uterine leiomyoma is associated with female sexual dysfunction in postmenopausal women. Yonsei Med J. 2019;60(8):791-5.

CHAPTER 14

Robotic-assisted Management of Fibroids

Indranil Dutta

■ INTRODUCTION

The integration of robotics into minimally invasive gynecological surgeries has revolutionized our treatment approaches. The availability of robotic technology has empowered us to refine our surgical techniques, achieving greater precision and safety levels than ever before.

Numerous technological advancements in robotics have significantly enhanced surgical capabilities. These include improved camera systems, which offer clearer visualization, enhanced depth perception, and the ability to minimize tremors. Additionally, robotics provide the potential for greater surgical precision and shorter learning curves compared to traditional laparoscopic methods.

In comparison to conventional laparoscopic surgeries, robotics consistently demonstrate superior surgical performance. It achieves this by minimizing operative time, reducing blood loss, and lowering the incidence of intra- and postoperative complications. Furthermore, the adoption of robotics has decreased the need to convert to abdominal surgery, offering patients a less-invasive treatment option with faster recovery times.

Overall, the utilization of robotics in gynecological surgeries represents a significant advancement, enabling surgeons to perform procedures with enhanced safety, precision, and efficiency.

ADVANTAGES OF LAPAROSCOPIC SURGERY

The transition to conventional laparoscopic or keyhole surgical approaches has brought numerous benefits to patients, as evidenced by various studies worldwide. These benefits primarily include a rapid recovery process and a quicker return to normal activities.[1] However, in surgeries requiring high precision, conventional laparoscopy can pose challenges due to restricted space and the complex anatomy of the pelvis.[2]

■ ROBOTIC SURGERY

The introduction of robotics has revolutionized surgical techniques by offering greater dexterity, intuitive movement, 3D visions, improved ergonomics, autonomy of camera control, and shorter learning curves.[3] Compared to conventional laparoscopy, robotic movements are filtered for tremors, and the camera system is secured and stabilized by the surgeon to provide an in-depth view of the tissues and operative field. While initially, 2D camera systems were popular, the realization that they lacked depth perception has led to the promotion of 3D systems.

Advantages and Drawbacks of Robotic Surgery

Robotic-assisted laparoscopy offers several advantages over conventional methods, including the ability of instruments to replicate the hand movements of the surgeon, unlike in conventional laparoscopy where hand and instrument movements are counterintuitive. The inclusion of a third arm allows for the safe placement of instruments when assistance is required. Additionally, robotics enable operations on obese patients with higher body mass index levels.[4]

However, robotic-assisted laparoscopy also has its drawbacks, including a lack of haptic feedback compared to conventional methods, the positioning of the surgeon away from the patient, and higher costs compared to conventional laparoscopic techniques.[5] Despite these limitations, the advantages of robotic-assisted laparoscopy make it a valuable tool in modern surgical practice.

STUDIES AROUND THE WORLD

A Cochrane review indicated that surgical complication rates were comparable between robotics and conventional methods in benign gynecological diseases.[6] However, several retrospective studies have shown that robotic-assisted laparoscopy improves surgical performance without increasing surgical time, blood loss, or intra- and postoperative complications.[7-9]

Despite the demonstrated benefits, the higher costs of robotic-assisted laparoscopy remain a significant disadvantage. However, it is important to note that costs are likely to decrease as surgical expertise increases.[10]

In light of these findings, it is essential for healthcare providers to offer patients a wide range of options by discussing the benefits and risks of each method of approach. This ensures that patients can make informed decisions about their treatment based on their individual needs and preferences.

FIBROIDS

Fibroids are among the most common benign tumors affecting women from reproductive age until menopause. Derived from smooth muscle cells of the myometrium, these tumors come in various types depending on their location, including subserosal, intramural, submucosal, and pedunculated fibroids. Ultrasonography is a straightforward diagnostic method for detecting fibroids.

Treatment options for fibroids range from medical management with medications such as combined hormonal contraceptives, GnRH analogs, or progestin-only pills to surgical interventions. Surgical treatments may include myomectomy or surgical removal of the uterus, depending on factors such as the patient's desire for fertility preservation or completion of their family. Surgical approaches can include open abdominal surgery or laparoscopic techniques.

In this context, the effective use of robotics in managing fibroids presents a promising avenue. However, it is important to note that robotic systems are not universally covered by insurance companies in many places, which poses a barrier to access. Once cost barriers are effectively addressed, robotics could potentially revolutionize the conservative management of fibroids, offering patients less-invasive treatment options with improved outcomes.

Procedure

The robotic approach is typically effective for fibroids measuring <15 cm or <15 myomas in total.[11] The patient is positioned in the dorsal lithotomy position, followed by tilting into the Trendelenburg position once trocars are secured. The assistant's port facilitates irrigation, suctioning, passing needles, tissue retraction, or morcellation. The fibroid is delineated and identified, and its extent is determined. Vasopressin may be injected into the fibroid as needed. In cases of myomectomy, an incision is made over the fibroid to enucleate it from the cavity using robotic tenaculums. Barbed sutures are utilized for closure of the scar area.[12]

For hysterectomy procedures, two Vicryl sutures are placed over the cervix, and a manipulator is introduced from below by an assistant to tightly secure the cervix. An abdominal Veress needle is introduced, followed by pneumoperitoneum and trocar placements. Bipolar diathermy is set at 40, and the uterus is identified and carefully manipulated using manipulators from below by an assistant. The round ligaments are identified and incised to expose the broad ligament. Step-by-step dissection is performed, and infundibulopelvic or round ligament pedicles are secured by bipolar or monopolar diathermy. The uterovesical fold is identified and carefully separated to expose the uterine arteries on either side and retract the urinary bladder. Further steps involve separating the uterus from tissues using bipolar or vessel sealer instruments. The cervix is identified, and dissection continues over the cervical cap placed with the manipulator. The uterus and tubes, with or without ovaries, are removed from the vagina or morcellated depending on feasibility. The vault is sutured with a continuous barbed suture. Hemostasis is achieved, and the procedure can be deemed complete with the withdrawal of instruments and ports. Ports are secured with sutures, and the patient can be discharged as early as possible the next day depending on her recovery pattern.

Robotic-assisted procedures offer advantages over conventional laparoscopy, providing surgeons with wider dexterity on the uterus, especially during myomectomy. The instruments enable surgeons to have a broader range of movements compared to traditional methods.

■ CONCLUSION

Robotics holds the potential to revolutionize the treatment of fibroids, offering a safer approach, improved outcomes, reduced blood loss, and shorter hospital stays. However, its widespread adoption in our country faces challenges due to cost considerations, availability of the system, and the learning curve involved.[13]

Systems like the Da Vinci System have already proven to be game-changers in the treatment of benign gynecological surgeries. Robotic myomectomy or hysterectomy stands as an equally effective and safe alternative in trained hands compared to traditional open or laparoscopic methods of surgery.

Nevertheless, further randomized studies are needed to solidify the benefits of robotic surgery, particularly in assessing long-term outcomes such as pregnancy, miscarriage, cesarean section rates, and birth rates in cases of myomectomy performed using robotics. Continued research and advancement in robotic technology will undoubtedly expand its applications and benefits in gynecological surgery.

■ REFERENCES

1. Walker JL, Piedmonte MR, Spirtos NM, Eisenkop SM, Schlaerth JB, Mannel RS, et al. Laparoscopy compared to laparotomy for comprehensive surgical staging of uterine cancer: Gynecologic Oncology Group LAP2 Study. J Clin Oncol. 2009;27(32):5331-6.

2. Hanna RK, Boggess JF. Applications of surgical robotics in gynecologic surgery. In: J Rosen, B Hannaford, R Satava (Eds). Surgical Robotics. Boston, MA: Springer; 2011. pp. 761-89.
3. Payne TN, Dauterive FR. A comparison of total laparoscopic hysterectomy to robotically assisted hysterectomy: surgical outcomes in a community practice. J Minim Invasive Gynecol. 2008;15(3):286-91.
4. Moss EL, Sarhanis P, Ind T, Smith M, Davies Q, Zecca M. Impact of obesity on surgeon ergonomics in robotic and straight-stick laparoscopic surgery. J Minim Invasive Gynecol. 2019;27(5):1063-9.
5. Schreuder HW, Verheijen RH. Robotic Surgery. BJOG. 2009;116(2):198-213.
6. Lawrie TA, Liu D, Dowswell T, Song H, Wang L, Shi G. Robot-assisted surgery in gynaecology. Cochrane Database Syst Rev. 2019;4:CD011422.
7. Lonnersford C, Persson J. Implementation and applications of robotic surgery within gynecologic oncology and gynecology: analysis of the first 1000 cases. Ceska Gynekol. 2013;78(1):12-9.
8. Patzkowsky KE, As-Sanie S, Advincula AP. Perioperative outcomes of robotic versus laparoscopic hysterectomy for benign disease. JSLS. 2013;17(1):100-6.
9. Smorgick N, Patzkowsky KE, Hoffman MR, Advincula AP, Song AH, As-Sanie S. The increasing use of robotic-assisted approach for hysterectomy results in decreasing rates of abdominal hysterectomy and traditional laparoscopic hysterectomy. Arch Gynecol Obstet. 2014;289(1):101-5.
10. Wright JD, Anath CV, Lewin SN, Burke WM, Lu YS, Neugut AI, et al. Robotically assisted vs laparoscopic hysterectomy among women with benign gynecologic disease. JAMA. 2013;309(7):689-98.
11. Quaas AM, Einarsson JI, Srouji S, Gargiulo AR. Robotic myomectomy: a review of indications and techniques. Rev Obstet Gynecol 2010;3(4):185-91.
12. Mahajan N, Moretti ML, Lakhi NA. Spontaneous early first and second trimester uterine rupture following robotic-assisted myomectomy. J Obstet Gynaecol. 2019;39(2):278-80.
13. Behera MA, Likes CE, Judd JP, Barnett JC, Havrilesky LJ, Wu JM, et al. Cost analysis of abdominal, laparoscopic and robotic assisted myomectomies. J Minim Invasive Gynecol 2012;19(1):52-7.

CHAPTER 15

Management of Recurrent Fibroids

Mridula Sharma

■ INTRODUCTION

The most prevalent benign tumor in premenopausal women is uterine fibroids, also known as leiomyomas. While 20–50% of women experience symptoms including abnormal uterine bleeding, pelvic pressure, discomfort, or bowel or urine issues, they are typically found accidentally by imaging in asymptomatic women.[1]

A few risk factors for the development of these benign tumors are age, Black ethnicity, family history, premenopausal status, and hypertension; contraceptive use, smoking in women with low body mass index, and low parity are protective factors, though.[1]

After a myomectomy, 15–33% of fibroids reappear, and within 5–10 years, 10–21% of women have a hysterectomy.[2,3] There is significant variation in the published rates and time to recurrence; they range from 12 to 15%, 31 to 43%, 51 to 62%, and 84% at 1, 3, 5, and 8 years, respectively.[4-6]

Although the exact biological source of uterine fibroids is uncertain,[7] genetic research indicates that they are monoclonal tumors.[8] The initiating event might be a mutation in myometrial stem cells HMGA2 or MED12.[9] Mature myometrial cells release paracrine proteins, like WNT ligands, in response to stimulation from estrogen and progesterone. These substances activate the β-catenin–T-cell transcription factor pathway by binding to the Frizzled receptor and causing the synthesis of transforming growth factor-β (TGF-β). This initiates proliferation via the Smad pathway in mutant cells. Therefore, it is likely that some mutant fibroid stem cells—which were too small to see or feel—were left behind during an open myomectomy. These fibroids have the potential to multiply exponentially over time and manifest symptoms due to de novo alteration of myometrial cells.

■ MANAGEMENT OF RECURRENT FIBROIDS

The management of recurrent uterine fibroids depends on various factors, including the severity of symptoms, the size and location of the fibroids, the patient's age, desire for future fertility, and overall health. Some common approaches to managing recurrent fibroids are:

- *Expectant management (observation):*
    - For small fibroids, not causing significant symptoms
    - Women is nearing menopause
    - Watch and Wait approach
    - Regular monitoring with ultrasound or other imaging techniques helps track fibroid growth and symptom progression
- *Medical management:*
    - *Hormonal therapy:* Hormonal medications can help manage fibroid-related symptoms **(Table 1)**.

TABLE 1: Hormonal therapy.

Drugs	Mechanism of action	Effect	Side effect
Combined oral contraceptive	• Ovulation inhibition • Inhibits release of sex steroids	• Reduces menstrual bleeding • Decreases growth of fibroid • Anemia correction	• Mastalgia • Headache Thromboembolism
Progestin-releasing intrauterine devices (IUDs)	Local progesterone release causes endometrial atrophy	Control heavy menstrual bleeding and may also reduce the size of fibroids	• Amenorrhea • Spotting per vaginum
Gonadotropin hormone-releasing hormone (GnRH) agonists	• When the activation of the GnRH receptors is prolonged, it causes desensitization followed by suppression of gonadotropin secretion • Initial flare response seen	Reduces the size of the fibroid in 50% of women within 3 months	• Bone demineralization. Give add-back therapy after 3–6 months of use • Fibroid regrowth on cessation of therapy
GnRH antagonists	Classical competitive blockage mechanism of GnRH receptors short onset of action and treatment duration No initial flare response	Decreases fibroid size by 40–50%, reduces menstrual blood loss in 77–84% of women by 6 months and 89% of women by 12 months of therapy	• Bone demineralization • Hypoestrogenic side effects

- *Selective progesterone receptor modulators (SPRMs):* The growth of leiomyoma is hormone-dependent, especially estrogens, and indeed, these tumors are a rarity before puberty and regress spontaneously after the menopause. Progesterone plays an enigmatic role by stimulating myoma growth through upregulating epidermal growth factor (EGF) and Bcl-2 expression; on the other hand, it is shown to inhibit growth through downregulation of insulin-like growth factor-1 (IGF-I) expression at the cellular level.[10]
    - *Mifepristone (MFP):* MFP, also named RU486, depicts the prototype surface plasmon resonance microscopy (SPRM), as clinically it was the first to be synthesized and utilized. Only three truly randomized controlled trials (RCTs) were found in a 2022 systematic Cochrane review,[11] that were done with MFP versus different medical therapies or any placebo, with 112 pariciapnts, who were given different dosages. It concluded that MFP relieves heavy menstrual bleeding, although it did not reveal any conclusive evidence for any effect on the volume of the fibroid. In two trials conducted in India, different schedules were used and evaluated; 50 mg was used in weekly/biweekly doses, leading to good results. The vaginal route for using 10 mg daily of MFP markedly reduced the volume of fibroids. Another meta-analysis, published in 2023,[12] considered 11 RCTs (using doses from 2.5

to 25 mg for 3–6 months and including 780 subjects). It showed opposite conclusion that MFP is effective in bringing down uterine and fibroid volume, taking care of hypermenorrhea, menstrual blood loss (MBL), and anemia, relieving pelvic pain, dysmenorrhea, and pelvic pressure. In Spain, a group concluded that a 5 mg dose was preferred to 10 mg.[13,14]

- *Ulipristal acetate (UPA):* It may be used for short-term treatment to control bleeding and shrink fibroids. Liver function should be monitored while on this medication. Most widely used and promising ulipristal acetate, code-named CDB-2914 or VA-2914, are available today. The study highlighted that UPA is effective in reducing fibroid volume and in controlling pain and bleeding, and it improves quality of life (QoL) of the patients, even when the treatment was discontinued.
- *Asoprisnil (ASP):* It is code-named J867, and the major metabolite is code-named J912. They are a class of progesterone receptor (PR) ligands having partial agonist and antagonist activities in vivo.[15] A multicentric RCT that used 5, 10, and 25 mg daily showed that ASP markedly suppressed the duration and intensity of uterine bleeding, leading to amenorrhea in a dose-associated manner (28%, 64%, and 83%), causing Hb concentration rise and decreasing volumes of fibroid and total uterus in the 25 mg group.
- *Proellex (Telapristone):* This SPRM has not been used much in the treatment of women having fibroids. It makes the endometrium inactive or atrophic with formation of cystic dilated glands. It causes secretory changes that coexist with mitoses and apoptotic bodies. On ultrasound, there was no hyperplasia; only increased thickness of endometrium was reported.[16]
- *Antiestrogens:* Goserelin brought down fibroid growth and endometrial thickness as compared with placebos. Fulvestrant did not bring much change in the fibroid volume or endometrial thickness or change endpoints such as endometrial histology or vaginal bleeding. An RCT compared the ability of the antiestrogen fulvestrant (as an intramuscular injection of 50, 125, or 250 mg) with that of the Gonadotropin Releasing Hormone Analogs (GnRHA) goserelin (as a subcutaneous injection of 3.6 mg), or an injection-matched placebo, once every 4 weeks, before hysterectomy, to reduce the growth of fibroid.[17]
- *Nonhormonal treatment:*
  - *Tranexamic acid:* This nonhormonal medication can reduce heavy menstrual bleeding. It is a synthetic derivative of lysine. It reversibly binds to five lysine-binding sites on plasminogen leading to inhibition of plasmin synthesis.
    Dose: 500 mg TDS (maximum for 5 days)
  - *Nonsteroidal anti-inflammatory drugs (NSAIDs):* They inhibit the synthesis of prostaglandins and reduce menstrual bleeding and dysmenorrhea.

Among the medical management of uterine fibroids, the most encouraging results are from the PR modulators and the orally active gonadotropin hormone releasing hormone receptor (GnRHR) blockers.

MINIMALLY INVASIVE PROCEDURES

- *Uterine artery embolization (UAE):* Uterine fibroid embolization is a popular treatment for uterine fibroids that generally has very good outcomes. This is a useful procedure for blocking the blood supply to fibroids, causing them to shrink.
- *MRI-guided focused ultrasound (MRgFUS):* Noninvasive ultrasound waves are used to destroy fibroids. Techniques like MRIgFUS surgeries have been available in recent times, which are approved by the Medicine Agency of the European Union (EMA) in the year 2002 and by the United States Food and Drug Administration (US-FDA) in the year 2004. This includes a noninvasive thermo-ablative technique, which combines anatomic details, visualization through MRI, with the therapeutic potential of high-intensity-focused ultrasound waves that can pass through the abdominal wall. It offers a clear three-dimensional anatomic resolution and thermal monitoring in real time. The procedure also provided the advantage of preserving fertility, in selected cases.
- *Laparoscopic radiofrequency ablation:* Radiofrequency energy is used to treat fibroids through laparoscopic surgery.[18]

SURGICAL OPTIONS

Recurrence of uterine fibroids is an indication for repeat surgery, if patient complains of:
- Abnormal uterine bleeding
- Dyspareunia/dysmenorrhea not responsive to medication
- Pelvic pressure
- Infertility
- Other symptoms, such as urinary problems, linked to fibroids

The rate of reoperation is lower after open myomectomy and is slightly higher after laparoscopic surgeries.
- *Myomectomy:* Surgical removal of fibroids while preserving the uterus, which is suitable for those who want to maintain fertility, can relieve bleeding and other symptoms in 80–90% of women. It is an option if the woman wants to preserve her uterus for another reason. The fibroids usually do not grow back after surgery, but new fibroids may develop. About 33% of women will be needing a repeat procedure for new fibroids within 5 years.

  This surgery is done depending on the number, size, and location of the fibroids.
  - *Hysteroscopy:* This has been found to be more effective for smaller and less number of fibroids. Hysteroscopy can also remove fibroids that have grown into the inside the body or cavity of uterus.
  - *Abdominal myomectomy:* This is better for large fibroids, but it usually leaves a bigger scar than the other two types.
  - *Laparoscopy:* This has a faster recovery period than abdominal myomectomy but needs finer expertise.
- *Hysterectomy:* It is an option if fibroids are many, large, and woman is not planning to have children. A few different ways are:
  - Abdominal hysterectomy
  - Vaginal hysterectomy
  - *Laparoscopic hysterectomy:* This procedure can also be done robotically. The surgeon may leave ovaries in place that will continue to produce female hormones.

- *Endometrial ablation:* This procedure destroys the uterine lining and can reduce menstrual bleeding associated with fibroids. Before the procedure, a pregnancy test and a test to check for endometrial cancer are performed. The intrauterine device (IUD) (if present) is removed. A procedure to thin the endometrial lining [dilatation and curettage (D&C)] may be performed. Different approaches, such as heat, electric current, microwave/radio wave energy, or freezing, can be used to destroy the endometrium. Temporary side effects from the procedure include cramps, vaginal discharge, and frequent urination. Risks and complications can be infection, bleeding, tearing of the uterine wall or bowel, and injury to surrounding organs.

Ongoing Monitoring

Regardless of the treatment chosen, regular follow-up is crucial to monitor the condition and assess any recurrence of fibroids or symptoms.

A few more points to consider regarding the management of recurrent uterine fibroids are as follows:

- *Second opinions:* It is entirely appropriate to seek a second opinion from another healthcare provider, especially if there are concerns for diagnosis or treatment plan. Another perspective can offer clarity and confidence in your decisions.
- *Clinical expertise:* Depending on the complexity of the case, one can seek care from a gynecologist who specializes in fibroids or a fibroid center. Specialized expertise can lead to more comprehensive and effective treatment.
- *Alternative medicine:* Some individuals explore complementary and alternative therapies such as acupuncture, herbal supplements, or dietary changes to manage fibroid symptoms. While these may provide relief for some, it is important to discuss them with the healthcare provider and ensure they will not interfere with prescribed treatment.
- *Family planning and pregnancy:* For women who want to become pregnant in the future, discussing fertility preservation options and family planning with a fertility specialist is essential. This can help ensure that any chosen treatment aligns with the reproductive goals.
- *Lifestyle modifications:* Maintaining a healthy lifestyle can help manage fibroid symptoms.
  - *Diet:* Have plenty of fruits and vegetables.
  - *Exercise:* Regular physical activity can help control weight and reduce symptoms.
  - *Stress management:* Stress reduction techniques like yoga or meditation may help alleviate symptoms.
  - Maintaining a healthy weight contributes to overall well-being.
- *Patient advocacy organizations:* There are patient advocacy organizations and online communities dedicated to fibroids. These can also provide valuable resources, give support, and provide connections with others going through similar experiences.
- *Long-term outlook:* While fibroids can be challenging to manage, many women find relief and successfully navigate their journey with the condition. Understanding that fibroids can be effectively managed can provide hope for a better quality of life.

■ CONCLUSION

The choice of treatment should be made in consultation with a healthcare provider, considering the specific circumstances and woman's preferences. It is important to discuss the goals, risks, and potential benefits of each option to make an informed decision. Additionally, staying up to date with the latest medical research and guidelines can help guide the treatment choices.

Remember that the choice of treatment should be individualized based on the patient's unique circumstances, including the severity of symptoms, desire for future fertility, and overall health.

■ REFERENCES

1. Kramer KJ, Ottum S, Gonullu D, Bell C, Ozbeki H, Berman JM, et al. Reoperation rates for recurrence of fibroids after abdominal myomectomy in women with large uterus. PLoS One. 2021;16(12):e0261085.
2. Singh SS, Belland L. Contemporary management of uterine fibroids: focus on emerging medical treatments. Curr Med Res Opin. 2015;31(1):1-12.
3. Reed SD, Newton KM, Thompson LB, McCrummen BA, Warolin AK. The incidence of repeat uterine surgery following myomectomy. J Womens Health (Larchmt). 2006;15(9):1046-52.
4. Yoo EH, Lee PI, Huh CY, Kim DH, Lee BS, Lee JK, et al. Predictors of leiomyoma recurrence after laparoscopic myomectomy. J Minim Invasive Gynecol. 2007;14(6):690-7.
5. Nezhat FR, Roemisch M, Nezhat CH, Seidman DS, Nezhat CR. Recurrence rate after laparoscopic myomectomy. J Am Assoc Gynecol Laparosc. 1998;5(3):237-40.
6. Fedele L, Parazzini F, Luchini L, Mezzopane R, Tozzi L, Villa L. Recurrence of fibroids after myomectomy: a transvaginal ultrasonographic study. Hum Reprod. 1995;10(7):1795-6.
7. Bulun SE. Uterine fibroids. N Engl J Med. 2013;369(14):1344-55.
8. Linder D, Gartler SM. Glucose-6-phosphate dehydrogenase mosaicism: Utilization as a cell marker in the study of leiomyomas. Science. 1965;150(3692):67-9.
9. Makinen N, Mehine M, Tolvanen J, Kaasinen E, Li Y, Lehtonen HJ, et al. MED12, the mediator complex subunit 12 gene, is mutated at high frequency in uterine leiomyomas. Science. 2011;334(6053):252-5.
10. Xu Q, Ohara N, Liu J, Amano M, Sitruk-Ware R, Yoshida S, et al. Progesterone receptor modulator CDB-2914 induces extracellular matrix metalloproteinase inducer in cultured human uterine leiomyoma cells. MHR: Basic Science of reproductive medicine. Mol Hum Reprod. 2008;14(3):181-91.
11. Tristan M, Orozco LJ, Steed A, Ramirez Morera A, Stone P. Mifepristone for uterine fibroids. Cochrane Database Syst Rev. 2012;2012(8):CD007687.
12. Shen Q, Hua Y, Jiang W, Zhang W, Chen M, Zhu X. Effects of mifepristone on uterine leiomyoma in premenopausal women: a meta-analysis. Fertil Steril. 2013;100(6):1722-6.
13. Carbonell JL, Acosta R, Pérez Y, Marrero AG, Trellez E, Sánchez C, et al. Safety and effectiveness of different dosage of mifepristone for the treatment of uterine fibroids: a double-blind randomized clinical trial. Int J Womens Health. 2013;5:115-24.
14. Esteve JL, Acosta R, Pérez Y, Rodriguez B, Seigler I, Sanchez C, et al. Mifepristone versus placebo to treat uterine myoma: a double-blind, randomized clinical trial. Int J Women's Health. 2013;5:361-9.
15. De Manno D, Elger W, Garg R, Lee R, Schneider B, Hess-Stumpp H, et al. Asoprisnil (J867): a selective progesterone receptor modulator for gynecological therapy. Steroids. 2003;68(10-13):1019-32.
16. Ioffe OB, Zaino RJ, Mutter GL. Endometrial changes from short-term therapy with CDB-4124, a selective progesterone receptor modulator. Mod Pathol. 2009;22(3):450-9.
17. Donnez J, Vivancos BH, Kudela M, Audebert A, Jadoul P. A randomized, placebo-controlled, dose-ranging trial comparing fulvestrant with goserelin in premenopausal patients with uterine fibroids awaiting hysterectomy. Fertil Steril. 2003;79(6):1380-9.
18. Kotani Y, Tobiume T, Fujishima R, Shigeta M, Takaya H, Nakai H, et al. Recurrence of uterine myoma after myomectomy: open myomectomy versus laparoscopic myomectomy. J Obstet Gynaecol Res. 2018;44(2):298-302.

Wandering Fibroids

Soniya Dhiman, Rishu Goel

■ INTRODUCTION

Uterine fibroids, known as leiomyomas, are benign tumors primarily composed of smooth muscle cells with varying amounts of fibrous connective tissue. These tumors are among the most common benign gynecological conditions in women of reproductive age, affecting 40-70% of women over the age of 30 years.[1] While the majority of women with uterine fibroids are asymptomatic, approximately 25% may experience symptoms such as pain or heaviness in the lower abdomen, abnormal uterine bleeding, or pressure symptoms depending on the fibroids' location. Management options include medical and surgical treatments, which are selected based on various factors such as size, site, presenting complaints, and feasibility of fibroid removal.

A distinct category of fibroids, *parasitic or wandering fibroids*, has been increasingly recognized, despite being known for over a century. These parasitic fibroids, classified by the International Federation of Gynecology and Obstetrics (FIGO) as type 8 fibroids along with cervical fibroids,[2] are unique because they have no direct attachment to the uterus. Instead, they can be located in various regions and receive their blood supply from adjacent structures. Parasitic fibroids are classified as primary when they arise from the detachment of pedunculated subserosal fibroids and as secondary when they occur after procedures such as laparoscopic hysterectomy or myomectomy, especially when morcellation has been used.

Parasitic fibroids can be asymptomatic and may be incidentally diagnosed during imaging or surgery for other indications, or they may present with a variety of symptoms depending on their location. Similar to uterine fibroids, parasitic fibroids are hormone-responsive. Although medical management has been attempted, surgical intervention remains the only definitive treatment option available to date. In this chapter, we will discuss this rare entity known as wandering or parasitic fibroids.

■ EPIDEMIOLOGY

Wandering fibroids are extremely rare. They were first described by Kelly and Cullens as "myomas that have, for some reason, become partially or almost completely detached from the uterus and receive their main blood supply from another source."[3] The evidence on parasitic myomas is limited to case reports and case series, with very few prospective and retrospective cohort studies available.[4] It was initially believed that morcellation during laparoscopic hysterectomy and myomectomy was the process by which these myomas originated. However, in a systematic review conducted by Van der Meulen et al., the overall incidence of parasitic myomas after laparoscopic surgeries was found to be between 0.12% and 0.95%, and after laparoscopic myomectomy, it was reported to be between 0.20% and 1.25%.[4]

■ PATHOGENESIS AND ETIOLOGY

Leiomyomas, the most common benign tumors in women of reproductive age, predominantly develop in the uterine corpus, typically arising from the myometrium. These tumors are hormone-dependent, responding well to sex steroid hormones such as estrogen and progesterone. As they grow, leiomyomas can extend either internally or externally, potentially becoming intramural, submucosal, or subserosal. Further external growth may lead to the development of pedunculated subserosal fibroids. Subserosal or pedunculated subserosal myomas may eventually outgrow their blood supply, leading to ischemic necrosis. To prevent this, the omentum may adhere to the peritoneal surface of the pedunculated myoma, providing the necessary blood supply. Over time, the pedicle may disappear, causing the myoma to become completely detached and parasitic, obtaining its blood supply from the omentum and other sources. These primary parasitic fibroids are very rare, with only a few case reports documented.[5,6]

The increasing number of case reports in the literature supports the theory that parasitic fibroids can develop due to the use of morcellation during laparoscopic myomectomy or hysterectomy. The first electrical cutting device for laparoscopic tissue removal from the abdominal cavity was introduced by Steiner et al.[7] During morcellation, small tissue fragments can disperse into the peritoneal cavity and regrow as parasitic myomas. The first case of a parasitic myoma following laparoscopic morcellation was reported in 1997 by Ostrzenski.[8] With the rising use of morcellation during laparoscopic procedures, the incidence of reported parasitic myomas has also increased. According to Cucinella et al., the estimated incidence ranges from 0.20% to 1.25%.[9]

Van der Meulen et al. conducted a systematic review of the literature to evaluate the risk factors and association of parasitic fibroids with morcellation. They concluded that morcellation appears to be a risk factor for the development of these rare tumors, which, like primary leiomyomas, are hormone-dependent. Exposure to sex steroids, such as hormone replacement therapy or pregnancy, is correlated with increased growth of these tumors.[4]

Huang et al. also demonstrated the estrogen dependency of parasitic myomas in a mouse model and highlighted the potential of hormonal manipulative therapies, including aromatase inhibitors (AIs), gonadotropin-releasing hormone (GnRH) agonists, and selective estrogen receptor modulators (SERMs), in managing wandering fibroids.[10]

Another theory explaining the pathogenesis of secondary parasitic leiomyomas considers the restricted vascular supply of the uterus as seen in uterine artery embolization or with the use of GnRH agonists. This vascular restriction forces the myoma to seek alternative, nonuterine sources of attachment and blood supply to continue growing.[3] Additionally, the de novo development of leiomyomas in extrauterine smooth muscles due to metaplastic changes has also been suggested, describing their occurrence in unexpected locations.[11]

■ VARIANTS OF PARASITIC LEIOMYOMA

The parasitic leiomyomas found in nonuterine locations can present in various forms with different clinical presentations. Due to their nonspecific signs and symptoms, diagnosing these fibroids can be challenging, and malignancy must be ruled out before confirming a diagnosis of parasitic leiomyoma. Imaging techniques such as ultrasonography, computed tomography (CT) scan, magnetic resonance imaging (MRI), and immunohistochemistry are crucial for confirming the diagnosis and ruling out malignancy. The various forms of these leiomyomas are discussed in the following text.

Parasitic Leiomyoma

Parasitic leiomyomas present as pelvic tumors separate from the uterus and are proposed to have clinical behaviors similar to uterine leiomyomas, including a similar theoretical response to treatment. They are typically found in the dependent parts of the abdominal cavity, including the intestines, peritoneum, omentum, port sites, and bladder flap, and receive their blood supply from these areas. Ultrasound whole abdomen and pelvis, CT, MRI, and positron emission tomography–computed tomography (PET-CT) help in making the diagnosis, whereas histopathology is confirmatory. Surgical removal is the definitive treatment for these fibroids.

Leiomyomatosis Peritonealis Disseminata

Leiomyomatosis peritonealis disseminata (LPD) presents with multiple peritoneal deposits on the subperitoneal surface of the uterus and other pelvic and abdominal viscera.[12] It is thought to result from multifocal peritoneal metaplasia. Although it can sometimes be confused with intravenous leiomyomatosis (IVL), LPD does not involve blood vessel invasion. Reports of LPD are rare, with only a few case reports and series published. For instance, Ye and Chen described LPD with low malignant potential in a woman with a history of laparoscopic myomectomy and hysterectomy.[13] Another case by Qin et al. reported LPD with pleural effusion after previous surgeries for uterine fibroids.[14] Hormones, specifically estrogen, are considered to be implicated in its pathogenesis, particularly observing their behavior in women with hormone replacement therapy, tamoxifen therapy, or during pregnancy. Associations of wandering fibroids with endometriosis have also been reported.[15] Diagnosis is challenging, and no definitive treatment exists; however, surgical removal is indicated, with medical management options such as hormone withdrawal therapy and treatments such as AIs, GnRH agonists, and estrogen inhibitors being considered in specific cases.

Intravenous Leiomyomatosis

Intravenous leiomyomatosis is an unusual benign form of parasitic leiomyoma first described by Marshall and Morris in 1959.[16] Two hypotheses are postulated to explain its etiopathogenesis. The first theory explains its origin from smooth muscle proliferation within vessels, leading to potential metastasis to distant sites. The second theory describes that there is a direct extension of the polypoidal projections into the muscular veins of the parametrium and broad ligament.[17] IVL is often suspected to be a uterine sarcoma, but histology showing benign smooth muscle cells distinguishes it from malignant lesions. In 50–75% of cases, IVL is confined to the parametrium and broad ligament, but it can extend to the inferior vena cava and right heart, leading to fatal outcomes. Association has also been reported with deep vein thrombosis.[18] Complete surgical removal with a multidisciplinary team is the only available treatment.

Benign Metastasizing Leiomyoma

Benign metastasizing leiomyoma (BML) consists of aggregates of smooth muscle cells located at sites such as the lung, abdominal cavity, retroperitoneum, muscular tissue, lymph nodes, blood vessels, or heart, with the lungs being the most common metastatic site.[19,20] These are usually found as incidental lung nodules and are believed to spread hematogenously from the uterus to distant sites.[21] Symptoms are often absent, though a small percentage of patients may experience respiratory issues if the lungs are involved.[22] Imaging with CT scans shows well-circumscribed nodular lesions, and PET-CT reveals absent fluorodeoxyglucose (FDG) uptake, differentiating BML from malignant lesions.

Before confirming BML, leiomyosarcoma and smooth muscle tumors of uncertain malignant potential (STUMP) must be ruled out.[23] Histological findings include well-differentiated spindle-shaped cells with low nuclear and cellular variance, no disorganized growth, and low mitotic figures. BML generally has a benign clinical course, remaining stable in number, size, and symptoms, though some cases report significant growth if untreated.[24]

As BML is hormone-dependent, hormonal manipulation via surgical (bilateral oophorectomy) or medical means (AIs, estrogen receptor blockers, and GnRH agonists) may be tried. Careful follow-up is necessary to monitor tumor regression or growth.

■ DIAGNOSIS

Parasitic fibroids vary widely in their presentation, typically depending on their location. The most common location is the pelvis. These typically present in late reproductive or premenopausal women, often with a history of surgery for uterine leiomyomas.[21]

Most of the time, parasitic fibroids present with nonspecific clinical signs and symptoms and are diagnosed incidentally during surgery for another reason. Abdominal pain is the most common presenting symptom (49%); other symptoms include heaviness or pressure depending on the fibroid's location. Larger fibroids can present as a palpable lump in the abdomen.[25] Other symptoms may include dysmenorrhea, abnormal uterine bleeding, dyspareunia, and, in some cases, acute abdomen.[26] For instance, a case of acute abdomen with a parasitic fibroid was reported where the detached fibroid was found attached to a fallopian tube, causing torsion and acute pain.[27] Symptoms can mimic adnexal mass torsion or present alongside other benign conditions such as endometrial cysts or endometriosis.[28] Depending on the fibroid's location, it can cause constipation (if located near the sigmoid colon) or urinary symptoms such as frequency, urgency, or retention if involving the urinary tract. Some case reports have shown that parasitic fibroids can present with features suggestive of malignancy, including ascites and elevated levels of tumor markers such as CA-125.[29]

A history of previous surgery, particularly hysterectomy or myomectomy involving power morcellation, can provide a clue toward diagnosing parasitic leiomyoma. However, cases have been reported where no previous surgical history was present, yet a final diagnosis of parasitic leiomyoma was made.[30]

Parasitic leiomyomas pose a diagnostic challenge due to their nonspecific presentation and variable locations. They can mimic other pelvic tumors, broad ligament cysts, or ovarian tumors. Their presence in unusual locations often raises suspicion of malignancy. For instance, LPD may present similarly to peritoneal carcinomatosis, and IVL may resemble renal cell carcinoma with tumor extension into the inferior vena cava. Benign metastasizing leiomyoma may be mistaken for lung or liver metastasis. Thus, when evaluating abdominopelvic masses, wandering or parasitic fibroids should be considered in the differential diagnosis. A newly diagnosed pelvic mass should be thoroughly investigated with physical examination and imaging techniques.

Transvaginal ultrasound can help differentiate them from ovarian masses. MRI can be useful in identifying the origin of the mass and distinguishing it from other pelvic tumors.[12] PET–CT helps differentiate from malignancy as parasitic fibroids show no FDG uptake.

Elevated tumor markers can complicate the diagnosis, and it is not surprising that parasitic fibroids are sometimes preoperatively diagnosed as malignant abdominopelvic tumors.[12] The combined knowledge of past surgical history, symptoms, and imaging can guide the diagnosis. The final diagnosis is made based on histology, where well-differentiated myocytes are present. Immunohistochemistry of lesions with antibodies against desmin, smooth muscle actin, vimentin, and caldesmon confirms mesenchymal derivation with smooth muscle differentiation of these tumors.

■ MANAGEMENT

A significant publication has highlighted a rising incidence of parasitic leiomyomas following endoscopic uterine surgeries, particularly those involving morcellation. Consequently, meticulous caution is paramount during the initial surgery. Various guidelines exist to mitigate the risk of iatrogenic parasitic fibroids. The use of a morcellation endo bag during power morcellation is recommended to prevent tissue spillage. Additionally, the American Association of Gynecologic Laparoscopists (AAGL) advocates for a thorough inspection and irrigation of the peritoneal cavity post procedure. Morcellation should be completely avoided if there is any suspicion of uterine malignancy.[31]

Management of parasitic leiomyomas involves surgical resection of the mass, which can be performed either via open or laparoscopic routes. The choice of surgical method depends on factors such as the size and location of the fibroids, the surgeon's expertise, and the availability of endoscopic surgery facilities. A multidisciplinary team approach is essential to ensure the complete resection of all tumors. During surgery, it is crucial to identify the vascular supply of the fibroid to prevent injury to adjacent structures. Surgical procedures may include debulking operations such as omentectomy, appendectomy, or bowel resection as necessary to remove fibroids from these areas.

Uterine myomas are hormone-dependent and respond well to various medical management options, including GnRH agonists, AIs, SERMs, progestins, and selective progesterone receptor modulators (SPRMs).[32] However, the role of medical treatments in managing parasitic fibroids is not well-established.

■ CONCLUSION

According to the FIGO classification system, parasitic or wandering fibroids are classified as type 8 fibroids. These fibroids have no direct attachment to the uterus and can be found in various body regions, receiving their blood supply from adjacent structures. Parasitic fibroids can be primary, arising from the detachment of pedunculated subserous fibroids, or secondary, developing after laparoscopic hysterectomy or myomectomy, particularly when morcellation is used.

They can be asymptomatic and are often diagnosed incidentally during imaging or surgery. Symptomatic cases may present with abdominal pain, pressure symptoms, dyspareunia, acute abdomen, and bowel or urinary symptoms, depending on the fibroid's location. Diagnostic modalities include ultrasonography, CT scan, MRI, and PET–CT, while histopathology and immunohistochemistry are used for definitive diagnosis. It is crucial to rule out malignancy, such as leiomyosarcoma, before confirming the diagnosis of parasitic fibroids. Surgery remains the mainstay of treatment.

REFERENCES

1. Bulun SE. Uterine fibroids. N Engl J Med. 2013;369:1344-55.
2. Munro MG, Critchley HO, Fraser IS, FIGO Menstrual Disorders Working Group. The FIGO classification of causes of abnormal uterine bleeding in the reproductive years. Fertil Steril. 2011;95(7):2204-8.e3.
3. Nezhat C, Kho K. Iatrogenic myomas: new class of myomas? J Minim Invasive Gynecol. 2010;17(5):544-50.
4. Van der Meulen JF, Pijnenborg JM, Boomsma CM, Verberg MF, Geomini PM, Bongers MY. Parasitic myoma after laparoscopic morcellation: a systematic review of the literature. BJOG. 2016;123(1):69-75.
5. Salih AM, Kakamad FH, Dahat AH, Habibullah IJ, Rauf GM, Najar KA. Parasitic leiomyoma: a case report with literature review. Int J Surg Case Rep. 2017;41:33-5.
6. Osegi N, Oku EY, Uwaezuoke CS, Alawode KT, Afolabi SA. Huge primary parasitic leiomyoma in a postmenopausal lady: a rare presentation. Case Rep Obstet Gynecol. 2019;2019:7683873.
7. Steiner RA, Wight E, Tadir Y, Haller U. Electrical cutting device for laparoscopic removal of tissue from the abdominal cavity. Obstet Gynecol. 1993;81:471-4.
8. Ostrzenski A. Uterine leiomyoma particle growing in an abdominal-wall incision after laparoscopic retrieval. Obstet Gynecol. 1997;89:853-4.
9. Cucinella G, Granese R, Calagna G, Somigliana E, Perino A. Parasitic myomas after laparoscopic surgery: an emerging complication in the use of morcellator? Description of four cases. Fertil Steril. 2011;96:e90-6.
10. Huang BS, Yang MH, Wang PH, Li HY, Chou TY, Chen YJ. Oestrogen-induced angiogenesis and implantation contribute to the development of parasitic myomas after laparoscopic morcellation. Reprod Biol Endocrinol. 2016;14(1):64.
11. Lalor PF, Uribe A, Daum GS. De novo growth of a large preperitoneal lipoleiomyoma of the abdominal wall. Gynecol Oncol. 2005;97(2):719-21.
12. Lete I, González J, Ugarte L, Barbadillo N, Lapuente O, Álvarez-Sala J. Parasitic leiomyomas: a systematic review. Eur J Obstet Gynecol Reprod Biol. 2016;203:250-9.
13. Ye Z, Chen L. Leiomyomatosis peritonealis disseminata with low-grade malignant change: a case report. Medicine (Baltimore). 2022;101(36):e30528.
14. Qin T, Wei L, Ma X, Qu H, Dang Y. Disseminated peritoneal leiomyoma associated with pleural effusion: a case description and literature analysis. Quant Imaging Med Surg. 2024;14(1):1266-71.
15. Toriyama A, Ishida M, Amano T, Nakagawa T, Kaku S, Iwai M, et al. Leiomyomatosis peritonealis disseminata coexisting with endometriosis within the same lesions: a case report with review of the literature. Int J Clin Exp Pathol. 2013;6:2949-54.
16. Marshall JF, Morris DS. Intravenous leiomyomatosis of the uterus and pelvis: case report. Ann Surg. 1959;149(1):126-34.

17. Chen J, Bu H, Zhang Z, Chu R, Qi G, Zhao C, et al. Clinical features and prognostic factors analysis of intravenous leiomyomatosis. Front Surg. 2023;9:1020004.
18. Li B, Chen X, Chu YD, Li RY, Li WD, Ni YM. Intracardiac leiomyomatosis: a comprehensive analysis of 194 cases. Interact Cardiovasc Thorac Surg. 2013;17(1):132-8.
19. Fan R, Feng F, Yang H, Xu K, Li S, You Y, et al. Pulmonary benign metastasizing leiomyomas: a case series of 23 patients at a single facility. BMC Pulm Med. 2020;20:292.
20. Pacheco-Rodriguez G, Taveira-DaSilva AM, Moss J. Benign metastasizing leiomyoma. Clin Chest Med. 2016;37(3):589-95.
21. Wu RC, Chao AS, Lee LY, Lin G, Chen SJ, Lu YJ, et al. Massively parallel sequencing and genome-wide copy number analysis revealed a clonal relationship in benign metastasizing leiomyoma. Oncotarget. 2017;8(29):47547-54.
22. Barnaś E, Książek M, Raś R, Skręt A, Skręt-Magierło J, Dmoch-Gajzlerska E. Benign metastasizing leiomyoma: a review of current literature in respect to the time and type of previous gynecological surgery. PLoS One. 2017;12(4):e0175875.
23. Hendrickson MR, Tavassoli FA, Kempson RL, et al. Mesenchymal tumours and related lesions. In: Tavassoli FA, Devilee P (Eds). World Health Organization Classification of Tumours: Pathology and Genetics of Tumours of the Breast and Female Genital Organs. Lyon, France: IARC Press; 2003. pp. 236-43.
24. Hoetzenecker K, Ankersmit HJ, Aigner C, Lichtenauer M, Kreuzer S, Hacker S, et al. Consequences of a wait-and-see strategy for benign metastasizing leiomyomatosis of the lung. Ann Thorac Surg. 2009;11:613-4.
25. Khan A, Shawl A, Leung PS. Parasitic leiomyoma of the greater omentum presenting as small bowel obstruction. J Surg Case Rep. 2018;2018(7):rjy164.
26. Pai AHY, Yen CF, Lin SL. Parasitic leiomyoma. Gynecol Minim Invasive Ther. 2020;9(2):108-9.
27. Vashistha P, Sharma M, Gupta B, Haq M. Wandering fibroid presented as acute abdomen: a rare case with diagnostic dilemma. J South Asian Feder Obstet Gynaecol. 2023;15(4):478-9.
28. Micha G, Galatis DG, Kalopita K, Strongylos A, Benekos C, Kalaitzi K, et al. Unusual case of a parasitic extra-uterine leiomyoma presenting with lower abdominal pain. Cureus. 14(10):e30141.
29. Wang YW, Fan Q, Qian ZX, Wang JJ, Li YH, Wang YD. Abdominopelvic leiomyoma with large ascites: a case report and review of the literature. World J Clin Cases. 2021;9(6):1424-32.
30. Al Manasra AR, Malkawi AS, Khammash MR. Parasitic leiomyoma. A rare cause of inguinal mass in females. Saudi Med J. 2011;32:633-5.
31. AAGL Advancing Minimally Invasive Gynecology Worldwide. AAGL practice report: morcellation during uterine tissue extraction. J Minim Invasive Gynecol. 2014;21:517-30.
32. Donnez J, Tatarchuk TF, Bouchard P, Puscasiu L, Zakharenko NF, Ivanova T, et al. Ulipristal acetate versus placebo for fibroid treatment before surgery. N Engl J Med. 2012;366:409-20.

CHAPTER 17

Cervical Fibroids

Aradhana Singh

■ INTRODUCTION

Cervical fibroids originate as benign smooth muscle tumors of uterine cervix. More commonly they are found as single subserous or interstitial myomas and rarely as submucosal or polypoidal myomas. Because of their anatomical positions they may compress urinary bladder and urethra anteriorly and rectum posteriorly. Treatment is mostly surgical and operating surgeon must be careful about preventing injuries to the surrounding pelvic structures during myomectomy or hysterectomy.

Incidence

Uterine fibroids are one of the most common benign smooth muscle tumors in women with a prevalence of 20–40% after the age of 35 years.[1,2] By menopause, up to 70% of women develop fibroids, but true incidence and prevalence are believed to be higher because most fibroids are asymptomatic and undiagnosed.[2] Only 25% of fibroids cause clinical symptoms and require intervention.[3] Ninety-five percent of leiomyomas are found in the uterine corpus[3] and cervical leiomyomas are rare with a frequency of only 0.6%.

■ ANATOMY

Cervical fibroids can arise from the supravaginal or vaginal portion of cervix. They can be interstitial or submucous and usually arise from the supravaginal part of the cervix and expands the cervix in all directions and displaces the uterine arteries and ureters laterally. During laparotomy, central cervical fibroids are usually seen as if the uterus is sitting on a huge cervical fibroid **(Fig. 1)**. Central supracervical fibroids can grow around the entire cervical canal and grow from the center displacing the ureters superiorly. Pedunculated cervical fibroids can arise from the endocervical canal and protrude through external os and even vaginal introitus. Sessile cervical fibroids arising from cervical lips around external cervical os are rare.[3]

Cervical fibroids can be classified as anterior, posterior, lateral, and central. Depending on their site, they produce clinical

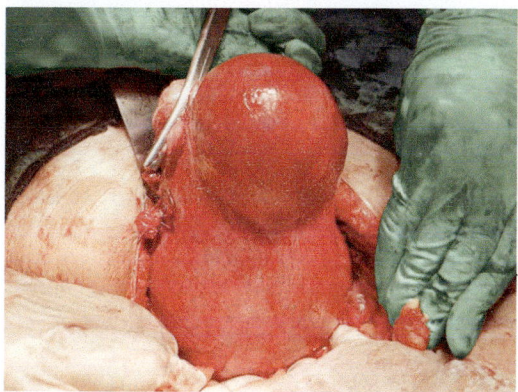

Fig. 1: Uterus sitting on a huge cervical fibroid.

symptoms.[4] Anterior cervical fibroids may push the bladder superiorly, while posterior fibroid bulges and flattens the pouch of Douglas. Lateral cervical fibroids expand into the broad ligament and compress the ureters laterally and superiorly. Their relation with ureters and uterine arteries is important as they always remain extracapsular.[5] Whatever may be the extent of displacement, this relation should be kept in mind while performing myoma surgery as it is an important safety feature. Central cervical fibroids expand the cervix in all directions and push the uterus upward **(Figs. 2 and 3)**. The uterus sits on an enlarged cervical fibroid, called a "Lantern on the top of St Paul's".[5]

■ SIGNS AND SYMPTOMS

Cervical fibroid may grow rapidly in some cases and cause various symptoms like pain due to obstruction of the cervix. A cervical fibroid can lead to infertility, urinary retention, increased urinary frequency, constipation, dysmenorrhea, menstrual irregularities, abnormal uterine bleeding (AUB), dyspareunia, feeling of pressure and heaviness in the pelvic region, and sometimes postcoital bleeding. Anterior fibroids cause pressure on the bladder and may lead to recurrent urinary tract infections while posterior fibroids lead to pressure symptoms on the bowel and constipation.[5]

■ DIAGNOSIS

The diagnosis of cervical myoma is by clinical examination. Pelvic examination may reveal a firm and abnormally enlarged cervix and sometimes a pulled-up cervix on per speculum examination. Imaging modalities like 3D pelvic ultrasound and magnetic resonance imaging (MRI) are done to define pelvic anatomy. The sonographic appearances of cervical myomas may vary from hypo- to hyperechoic, depending on the ratio of smooth muscles to connective tissue. Calcification and degeneration can also be identified on ultrasound. Leiomyomas have a typical vascular pattern on color Doppler ultrasound, showing a peripheral rim of vascularity from which few vessels penetrate the center of the tumor.

MRI imaging may be required to identify the distorted cervical anatomy and determine the extent of cervical myoma. It helps assess the accurate size, position, extent, and number of myomas. MRI differentiates adenomyosis from myomas and helps

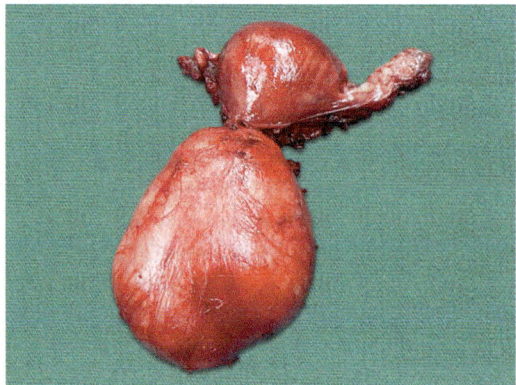

Fig. 2: Huge cervical fibroid expending the cervix in all directions—posterior view.

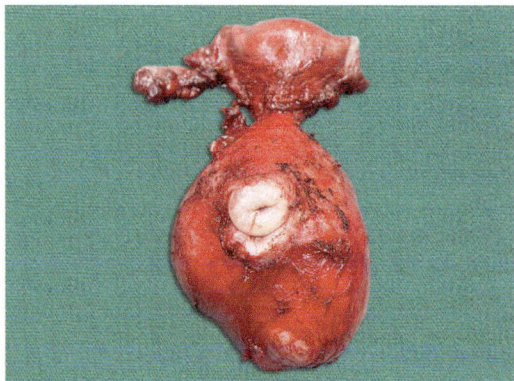

Fig. 3: Huge cervical fibroid expending the cervix in all directions—anterior view.

in planning the surgery or conservative management of these conditions.

TREATMENT

Expectant Management

Expectant management is advantageous in asymptomatic women with small fibroids or those who do not want any intervention. Women experiencing symptoms need to be treated with either medical, surgical, or other conservative modalities like uterine artery embolization (UAE).[6]

Medical Management

- For short-term therapy, gonadotropin-releasing hormone (GnRH) analogs are required for AUB associated with LM. They can be used with or without add-back therapy. An oral GnRH antagonist along with hormonal add-back therapy can also be considered for AUB-L.
- Tranexamic acid can be considered for AUB-L.

Uterine Artery Embolization

Uterine artery embolization is done to reduce the size of myoma when it is very small or surgery is to be postponed for some time. It can also be done as a preoperative procedure to reduce the size of fibroid. UAE is recommended for women with symptomatic fibroids who wish to keep their uterus, but they should be counseled about the limited data on reproductive outcomes.[6,7]

Surgical Management

The most common therapy for cervical myomas is surgery, which is challenging because of their difficult anatomical locations and close proximity with ureters, bladder, and bowel. There is a risk of intraoperative hemorrhage. Central cervical fibroid can be seen compressing lateral pelvic structures **(Figs. 4 and 5)**. Cervical leiomyoma poses difficulty while performing fertility-preserving surgery and requires skills of an experienced surgeon. Standard surgical approaches to cervical myomas are still lacking and depend on factors such as size, type, numbers, choice of patients regarding fertility preservation, and expertise of surgeons. Intervention radiology procedures are also performed for patients who wish to preserve their uterus.

For removing a large cervical fibroid, there are some important anatomical relations to

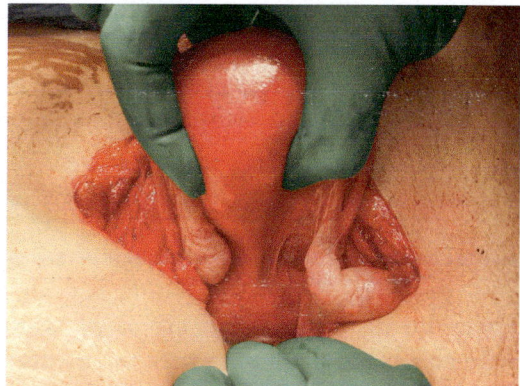

Fig. 4: Central cervical fibroid compressing lateral pelvic structures.

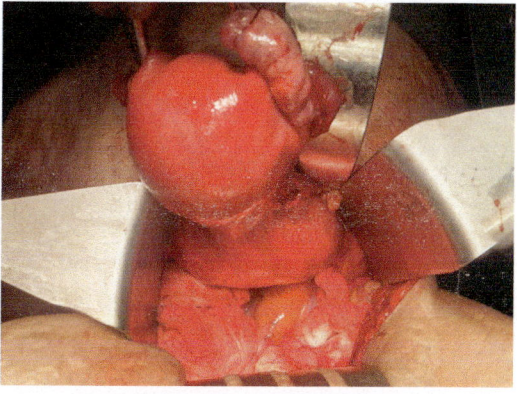

Fig. 5: The uterus sitting on an enlarged cervical fibroid, like a "Lantern on the top of St Paul's".

be kept in mind. The anatomical distortions that are to be kept in mind to avoid injury to the uterine vessels, ureter, and bladder, are:[8]
- Upward and outward displaced uterine vessels
- Pulled-up bladder
- Laterally and upward displaced uterus.

Enucleation of a large cervical myoma followed by total abdominal hysterectomy and bilateral salpingectomy has been reported.[9] Injury to the ureter can be avoided with preoperative cystoscopy-guided bilateral ureteral stenting, intraoperative tracing of the ureter before applying a clamp, and dissection inside the fibroid capsule. Sometimes, the lateral cervical fibroid has to be enucleated intraoperatively while performing hysterectomy to create space in the pelvic cavity and identify the course of ureter **(Fig. 6)**.

A study of 16 cases of cervical myomectomy performed safely by developing a uniform strategy and fixed surgical steps was done by Shozo Matsuoka et al.[10] Even during laparotomy, six steps were followed: (1) Attempt to reduce the myoma size by preoperative GnRH injections, (2) determining the anatomical relationship of myoma with the surrounding organs, (3) temporary blocking the uterine artery flow by using vessel clips, (4) suppressing the bleeding with intraoperative vasopressin use, (5) giving incision over myometrium to avoid damaging the surrounding structures, and (6) while suturing the myoma bed, the bottom of the wound should be pulled up by forceps to avoid formation of dead space.[10] Intraoperative identification of the ureters and preoperative ureteric stenting are the important precautions to avoid ureteric injuries. Intracapsular enucleation of the fibroid is a safer way to avoid ureteric injuries during surgery.

CONCLUSION

Cervical fibroids are difficult to diagnose and treat because of their varied presentations and pelvic location. Meticulous clinical examination along with various imaging modalities like ultrasound and MRI helps in diagnosing cervical fibroids. While managing surgically, the expertise of a surgeon is crucial in managing cervical fibroids safely. The careful identification of laterally displaced ureters and prevention of injuries to the urinary bladder and ureter are important during surgery. Dissection and enucleation of the cervical fibroid are required when fertility preservation is desired.

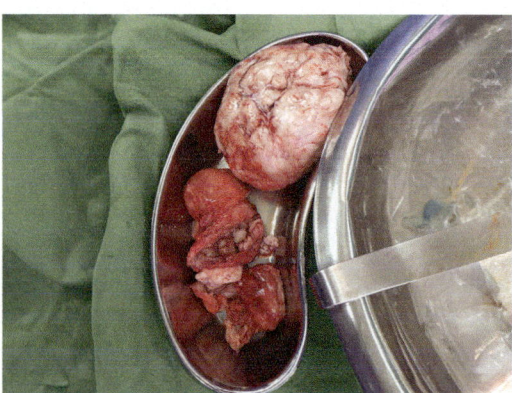

Fig. 6: Anterolateral cervical fibroid, enucleated while performing hysterectomy.

REFERENCES

1. Kaushal A, Kaur M, Bhalla V, Kaur D. Unusual giant central cervical leiomyoma: Surgical challenge. Int J Reprod Contracept Obstet Gynecol. 2018;7(12):5197-200.
2. Tiltman AJ. Leiomyomas of the uterine cervix: A study of frequency. Int J Gynecol Pathol. 1998;17(3):231-4.
3. Singh S, Chaudhary P. Central cervical fibroid mimicking as chronic uterine inversion: A case report. Int J Reprod Contracept Obstet Gynecol. 2013;2(4):687-8.
4. Moher D, Liberati A, Tetzlaff J, Altman DG; PRISMA Group. Preferred reporting items for

systematic reviews and meta-analyses: the PRISMA statement. BMJ 2009;339:b2535.
5. Ferrari F, Forte S, Valenti G, Ardighieri L, Barra F, Esposito V, et al. Current treatment options for cervical leiomyomas: a systematic review of literature. Medicina (Kaunas). 2021;57(2):92.
6. Hu J, Tao X, Yin L, Shi Y. Successful conservative treatment of cervical pregnancy with uterine artery embolization followed by curettage: a report of 19 cases. BJOG 2016;123(Suppl 3):97-102.
7. American College of Obstetricians and Gynecologists. (2021). ACOG updated guidelines on uterine fibroids-Available from https:// www.acog.org/womens-health/faqs/uterine-fibroids [Last accessed June, 2024].
8. Takeuchi H, Kitade M, Kikuchi I, Shimanuki H, Kumakiri J, Kobayashi Y, et al. A new enucleation method for cervical myoma via laparoscopy. J Minim Invasive Gynecol. 2006;13(4):334-6.
9. Mujalda A, Kaur T, Jindal D, Sindhu V, Jindal P, Mujalda J. Giant cervical fibroid: a surgical challenge. Cureus 2023;15(5):e39602.
10. Matsuoka S, Kikuchi I, Kitade M, Kumakiri J, Kuroda K, Tokita S. Strategy for laparoscopic cervical myomectomy. J Minim Invasive Gynecol. 2010;17(3):301-5.

CHAPTER 18: Uterine-preserving Treatment Modalities

Apurba Kumar Dutta

INTRODUCTION

Uterine fibroids (also known as leiomyomas or myomas) are benign tumors, originating from uterine smooth muscles. These are the most common benign tumors in the reproductive age group of women.[1,2] They may cause menorrhagia, metrorrhagia, polymenorrhagia, and other abnormal uterine bleeding resulting in low hemoglobin, chronic pelvic pain, subfertility, and recurrent abortions. Sometimes, they may be asymptomatic.

Surgical therapies are curative in symptomatic cases, but medical treatments may consider first-line therapy for fertility preservation and postponed or delay surgery. This chapter discusses all the treatment modalities for the preservation of the uterus in symptomatic fibroids.

Most fibroids are asymptomatic and do not need any intervention; they just need follow-up to record the size and growth of the fibroid.

For symptomatic uterine fibroids, treatment options include medical, radiologically guided interventions, and finally surgery. Women's treatment goals, efficacy, safety profile, and need for repeat interventions should be considered.

In past, surgical interventions were considered the only definitive treatment for uterine fibroids, but medical, nonsurgical, and surgical treatments for fertility preservation and delayed invasive surgeries, with good efficacy and fewer side effects, are now available.

COMBINATION ORAL CONTRACEPTIVES

Various studies conclude that the use of combined oral contraceptives (COCs) can lead to a significant reduction in uterine blood flow in women with symptomatic fibroids.[3] Since fibroid growth is initiated by estrogens and progestins, COCs were thought to stimulate fibroid growth. But recently, a meta-analysis concluded that oral contraceptives are not a contraindication for use in the treatment of symptomatic fibroid.[4] COCs improve heavy uterine bleeding in symptomatic fibroids when used for a short term. They have a negative effect on the proliferation of endometrium but do not help in reducing the uterine size or volume of uterine fibroid.[3,4]

Progestins

Progestins are used in a cyclic manner for bleeding control in abnormal uterine bleeding without any structural defects, like in the case of bleeding associated with endometrial hyperplasia or perimenopausal menorrhagia. However, like COCs, some do not recommend the use of progestin in treating symptoms caused by uterine fibroids.[5] In some studies, medroxyprogesterone acetate (DMPA) injection is given to patients having abnormal uterine bleeding due to fibroid.[6] 6 months after injection, it induced amenorrhea in 30% cases, 70% of patients found significant reduction in bleeding, and 15% had improved in hemoglobin and hematocrit. Radiologically, the size of uterus and uterine fibroid volumes reduced by 48% and 33% of the total, respectively. Few other studies were conducted to assess the efficacy of progestins orally in patients with uterine fibroids. One study was conducted to determine lynestrenol versus oral progestogen versus leuprolide, which is a gonadotropin hormone-releasing hormone (GnRH) agonist. This study shows no appreciable improvement in pelvic pain and uterine bleeding associated with fibroids. Treatment of fibroids with progestins may be beneficial, but may cause histopathological changes, a raise in cellularity, and an increase in mitotic activity and can mimic leiomyosarcoma and tumors of smooth muscle.

Levonorgestrel-releasing Intrauterine System

In 2009, the Food and Drug Administration (FDA) approved the levonorgestrel-releasing intrauterine system (LNG-IUS) for the treatment of heavy menstrual bleeding for women who also opt for intrauterine devices for contraception. Zapata et al.[7] found a reduction in menstrual blood loss in 11 studies which they included in the analysis. They also found an appreciable increase in ferritin level, hematocrit, and hemoglobin. Many studies demonstrated a significant reduction in menstrual flow as well as hemoglobin levels in women with uterine fibroids associated with abnormal uterine bleeding. However, they failed to demonstrate a significant change in the size of the uterus and volume of the fibroid.[8–10]

Gonadotropin Hormone-releasing Hormone Agonists

Native GnRH, which is a decapeptide, is produced and released from the hypothalamus in a pulsatile pattern. GnRH agonists are synthetic decapeptides structurally similar to the natural GnRH, but these are more potent having a longer half-life compared to native GnRH[11,12] When administered, initially they increase the secretion of follicle-stimulating hormone (FSH) and luteinizing hormone (LH), also known as "flare effect." After the initial flare effect, they cause downregulation of receptors, followed by a hypogonadotropic hypogonadal state 1–3 weeks later, known as "pseudomenopause." As we know leiomyoma growth is initiated and stimulated due to estrogen. This hypogonadotropic hypogonadal state leads to hypoestrogenic, which is responsible for the pharmacologic effect of GnRH agonists. Cochrane reviewed 26 trials to demonstrate the effectiveness of GnRH agonists before myomectomy or hysterectomy and showed significant improvement in symptoms.[13] There is a notable increase in the preoperative as well as postoperative levels of hemoglobin. It also helps in a significant reduction in the size and volume of the uterus as well as myomas and stay in the hospital. However, after long-term use, it causes menopausal symptoms, such as hot flashes and atrophic vaginitis. It also reduces bone mineral density (BMD). Thus, GnRH agonists are mainly used for less duration and as adjuvant therapy. Due to these hypoestrogenic side effects, hormonal add-back therapy is necessary for long-term GnRH agonist therapy to counter hypoestrogenic symptoms and preserve BMD.[14,15]

Treatment with GnRH agonists may cause changes in histopathology of fibroids and complicate the surgical procedure. Preoperative use of leuprolide acetate causes degeneration of myomas. It also obliterates the interface between the myometrium and myoma (Capsule), causing difficulty in the enucleation and removal of myomas. Pretreatment also results in reduction in the size of fibroids, making them more soft and thus hard to find during myomectomy. Thus, fibroids may be missed during surgery.

Gonadotropin Hormone-releasing Hormone Antagonists

Gonadotropin hormone-releasing hormone antagonists inhibit the release of FSH and LH immediately by suppressing GnRH receptors at pituitary. This leads to a decrease in estradiol levels. The hypoestrogenic state helps in improving bleeding patterns and also reduces the size of the uterine fibroid. Its effects started within 3 weeks after starting the therapy.[16,17] Due to its faster action, and practically no gonadotropin side effects like flare and faster relief of symptoms, it is well tolerated by patients.[18]

Selective Progesterone Receptor Modulators

Selective progesterone receptor modulators are the molecules having tissue-specific effects at progesterone receptors (PRs). They have multiple effects. It can be a PR antagonist or agonist or both.[19] Mifepristone, onapristone, telapristone, ulipristal, and asoprisnil are very effective treatments for fibroids. Among SPRMs, mifepristone was the one used first in clinical practice in three decades. It has PR antagonistic properties.[20-22] Most of the initial clinical studies on SPRMs use mifepristone and asoprisnil.[22-24] Both of them significantly reduce uterine fibroid size and other myoma-associated symptoms. Ulipristal acetate (UPA) is a new SPRM agent, which is approved by FDA as an emergency contraceptive. UPA underwent clinical trials and was found to significantly lower myoma size and volume, reduce bleeding, and induce amenorrhea.[25,26]

Selective Estrogen Receptor Modulators

Selective estrogen receptor modulators (SERMs) are nonsteroidal estrogen receptor (ER) ligands having tissue-specific either ER agonist or antagonist properties. They act by alterations in gene expression and are tissue-specific. They are originally used for adjuvant therapy in ER-positive breast cancer. Tamoxifen and raloxifene are two commonly studied SERMs for the treatment of myomas.[27-29]

Aromatase Inhibitors

Aromatase inhibitors block the conversion of androgens to estrogens extragonadally. They are widely used as an adjuvant therapy with ER-positive breast cancer in postmenopausal women. They are able to inhibit estrogen production.[30-32] These properties make AI ideal molecules for treating fibroids. They are as effective as GnRH analogs in reducing uterine myoma volume and other symptoms without compromising the level of estrogen.

Letrozole (2.5 or 5 mg daily) and Anastrazole 1 g daily are the most common AIs studied for myoma treatments.[31-33] Many observational studies conclude a significant reduction in uterine fibroid size and improvement of symptoms with AI treatment. Several small observational studies have shown a reduction in fibroid size and improvement of symptoms with AI therapy.

A Cochrane review of one study concluded that there are insufficient data to support the therapeutic use of AIs for women with symptomatic fibroids.

UTERINE-PRESERVING SURGICAL MODALITIES

Current management of fibroids includes mostly surgical interventions.

Though ideal therapy depends on the woman's age, it is wise to retain her fertility and delay or avoid radical interventions like hysterectomy.

Uterus preserving procedures include:
- Hysteroscopic myomectomy
- Laparoscopic or open (laparotomy) myomectomy
- Uterine artery embolization (UAE)
- Ultrasound or radiological-guided procedures

Hysteroscopic Myomectomy

There are several alternative procedures based on the experience of the operating surgeon and the availability of equipment.

Most commonly pedunculated fibroids are removed with laser fiber or the resectoscope (loop).

The second alternative is a one-step technique, where the complete excision of fibroids is done in a single step by the slicing technique. Myoma cuts into small pieces. The procedure is considered to be finished on visualization of myometrial fasciculate fibers.

In a third procedure, removal of the myoma is done in two steps [International Federation of Gynecology and Obstetrics (FIGO) classification type 1–3 fibroid]. In the first step, there is ablation or resection of the protruded part of the myoma, and the remaining intramural component migrates into the uterine cavity, which allows safe and complete excision of the myoma during the second step.

Hysteroscopic myomectomy is definitely effective in controlling symptoms like bleeding, but failures are reported like parasite fibroids, adenomyosis, or partial removal of big intramural myomas.

Laparoscopic Myomectomy

Laparoscopic myomectomy has many advantages: Postoperative morbidity is very low and recovery is fast. Moreover, no difference in the pregnancy rate or its outcomes following laparoscopic versus abdominal myomectomy is observed (laparotomy).

About 10 mm and 2–3.5 mm ancillary ports are usually used. A transversal or vertical (longitudinal) incision is made depending on the site of the myoma. A classically unipolar hook is utilized, and other modalities like CO_2 laser for myomectomy are also used. Preoperatively uterine artery ligation and intraoperatively injection vasopressin are useful to lessen the bleeding during operation.

Morcellators are used to remove myomas; some gynecologists also remove vaginally through the pouch of Douglas or maybe through a small incision below the umbilicus to reduce the risk of the spread of specimen pieces while doing morcellation.

Many used bag morcellation to minimize the risk of tissue spread; data are lacking to suggest that bag morcellation will reduce the complications in the postoperative period.

Laparoscopic Cryomyolysis and Thermocoagulation

Cryomyolysis and thermocoagulation are based on the principle of suppression and reduction of main vasculature and induce shrinkage of fibroids through sclerohyaline degeneration (either by very high or by very low temperatures).

Cryomyolysis: In this technique, a cryoprobe is put inside the fibroid and reduces the temperature to <−90°C.

Laparoscopic thermocoagulation: In this technique, bipolar and monopolar probes are put inside the fibroid and then electrical current is delivered. Recently, laser (YAG) has been used successfully in place of electric current. The major drawback is the unavailability of the specimen for histological evaluation.

Uterine Artery Occlusion

Occlusion of the main arterial supply, that is, uterine arteries, can be tried but found to have similar results as in vaginal occlusion. Moreover, the outcomes following treatment are inferior with respect to myoma size reduction and devascularization as compared to UAE.

ALTERNATIVES TO SURGICAL INTERVENTION

Uterine Artery Embolization

Uterine artery embolization is used as therapy for symptomatic uterine myomas in patients who want to preserve their fertility. It was first used in 1995.

As the name suggests, in UAE, there is occlusion of uterine artery causing ischemic necrosis of the uterine fibroids. Almost all fibroids are targeted at the same time. In randomized controlled trials, the results following UAE are similar in terms of quality of life (QoL) to that achieved post surgery, with additional benefits of short hospital stay as well as earlier return to normal activities.

Uterine artery embolization is highly efficient in reducing symptoms such as a significant decrease in uterine bleeding and reduction of the size of the fibroid. The major drawbacks are returning of symptoms and chances of operation or procedure again: 15–20% after the complete procedure and up to 50% in the case of an incomplete procedure.

Other complications include:
- *Pain in abdomen:* UAE cases of ischemic degeneration of fibroids
- Infection
- *Ovarian reserve:* Ovarian reserve is reduced after UAE. Many studies conclude that reduction in ovarian reserve may happen in patients of age 45 years or more.

Recently, emphasized that UAE is a relative contraindication in women's desire for future pregnancy, as there is a lack of data that ensure good fertility outcomes. One RCT compared UAE with myomectomy. There were more favorable outcomes following surgical removal compared to UAE-abortion rate (23% vs. 64%), positive pregnancy rate (78% vs. 50%), and delivery rate (48% vs. 19%).

Magnetic Resonance-guided Focused Ultrasound

High-frequency magnetic resonance-guided focused ultrasound surgery (MRgFUS). It is based on thermal ablation of myomas by visualizing the exact site through MRI. After the localization of myoma, ultrasonic energy is pointed into the fibroid which induces coagulative tissue necrosis. Theoretically, there is minimal injury to near tissues but injury to neighboring structures occurs.

Reviewed that hyperintensive images on MRI as compared to hypointensive images of fibroids reduced the success rate of treatment.

Major limitations of MRgFUS:
- Very few patients with symptomatic fibroids are eligible for MRgFUS.
- Pregnancy outcome following MRgFUS is compromised compared to surgery.

Uterine-preserving Treatment Modalities

- Costly procedure
- *Treatment failure:* Approximately 30% of the women who underwent MRgFUS need additional treatment like surgery.

There is paucity of data on the above treatment and further RCT and data are required to determine the safety and adverse effects of the treatment.

Postprocedure MRI and prediction mapping based on MRI and screening are very important to assess the therapeutic responses and help in reducing failure of therapy. Many trials found more complication rate in pregnancy following MRgFUS treatment.

Vaginal Occlusion of the Uterine Arteries

In this technique, a device similar to a clamp is used to occlude uterine artery for 6 hours. It leads ischemia to fibroid by stopping uterine blood supply. For women wishing to preserve their fertility, this procedure is not recommended.

Demonstrated reduction in myoma volume by one-fourth and in uterine bleeding by half. For this technique too, data are insufficient with big populations. More researches are required to establish the effectiveness and safety of the procedure.

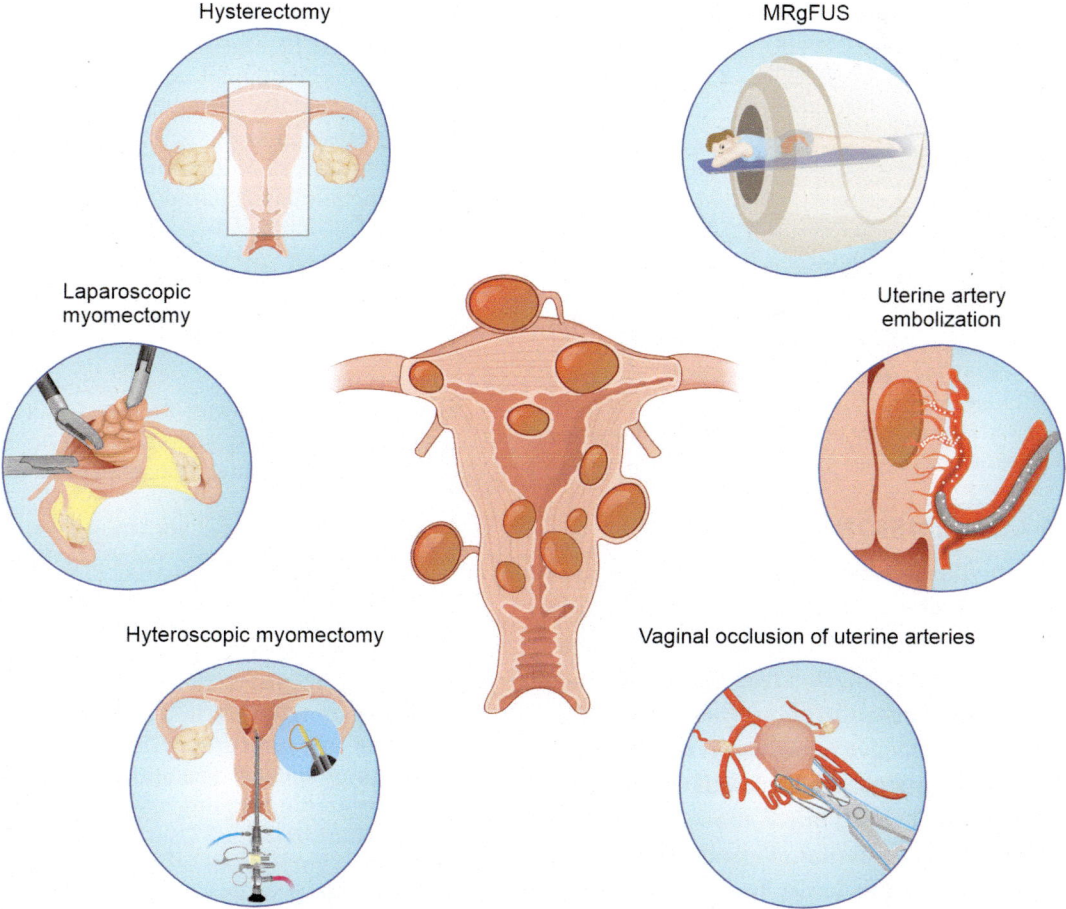

Fig. 1: Uterus-preserving treatment modalities.

UTERUS-PRESERVING TREATMENT MODALITIES (FIG. 1)

- Medical therapy:
  - OCPs:
    - Progestins
    - LNG-IUS
    - GnRH agonist
    - GnRH antagonist
    - SPRMs
    - SERMs
    - AIs
- Surgical
  - Myomectomy
    - Hysteroscopy
    - Laparoscopy
    - Laparotomy
  - Laparoscopic
    - Cryomyolysis
    - Thermocoagulation
  - Uterine artery occlusion
    - Laparoscopy
    - Vaginally
- Nonsurgical
  - UAE
  - MRgFUS

(AIs: Aromatase inhibitors; MRgFUS: magnetic resonance-guided focused ultrasound surgery; OCPs: oral contraceptive pills; LNG-IUS: levonorgestrel-releasing intrauterine system; GnRH: gonadotropin hormone-releasing hormone; SERMs: selective estrogen receptor modulators; SPRMs: selective progesterone receptor modulators; UAE: uterine artery embolization)

CONCLUSION

Uterine fibroids are common benign tumors in women of reproductive age. Asymptomatic uterine fibroids do not require any treatment. With delay in childbearing, more women require fertility-preserving treatments. The patient should give information regarding all treatment options (medical, radiological, and surgical) and which one is most appropriate and which one is not. Various modalities are currently available, but some require more investigation to establish efficacy and safety profile. The treatment of choice is based on the women's prime aim of the therapy, effectiveness of the treatment, safety profile, and need of repeated interventions.

REFERENCES

1. Linder D, Gartler SM. Glucose-6-phosphate dehydrogenase mosaicism: Utilization as a cell marker in the study of leiomyomas. Science. 1965;150:67-9.
2. Holdsworth-Carson SJ, Zaitseva M, Vollenhoven BJ, Rogers PA. Clonality of smooth muscle and fibroblast cell populations isolated from human fibroid and myometrial tissues. Mol Hum Reprod. 2014;20:250-9.
3. Marret H, Fritel X, Ouldamer L, Bendifallah S, Brun JL, De Jesus I, et al. Therapeutic management of uterine fibroid tumors: Updated French guidelines. Eur J Obstet Gynecol Reprod Biol. 2012;165:156-64.
4. Qin J, Yang T, Kong F, Zhou Q. Oral contraceptive use and uterine leiomyoma risk: a meta-analysis based on cohort and case-control studies. Arch Gynecol Obstet. 2013;288:139-48.
5. Hoffman BL, Williams JW. Williams Gynecology, 2nd edition. New York: McGraw-Hill Medical; 2012.
6. Venkatachalam S, Bagratee JS, Moodley J. Medical management of uterine fibroids with medroxyprogesterone acetate (Depo Provera): a pilot study. J Obstet Gynaecol. 2004;24:798-800.
7. Zapata LB, Whiteman MK, Tepper NK, Jamieson DJ, Marchbanks PA, Curtis KM. Intrauterine device use among women with uterine fibroids: a systematic review. Contraception. 2010;82:41-55.
8. Socolov D, Blidaru I, Tamba B, Miron N, Boiculese L, Socolov R. Levonorgestrel releasing-intrauterine system for the treatment of menorrhagia and/or frequent irregular uterine bleeding associated with uterine leiomyoma. Eur J Contracept Reprod Health Care. 2011;16:480-7.
9. Jiang W, Shen Q, Chen M, Wang Y, Zhou Q, Zhu X, et al. Levonorgestrel-releasing

intrauterine system use in premenopausal women with symptomatic uterine leiomyoma: a systematic review. Steroids. 2014;86:69-78.
10. Kriplani A, Awasthi D, Kulshrestha V, Agarwal N. Efficacy of the levonorgestrel-releasing intrauterine system in uterine leiomyoma. Int J Gynaecol Obstet. 2012; 116:35-8.
11. Islam MS, Protic O, Giannubilo SR, Toti P, Tranquilli AL, Petraglia F, et al. Uterine leiomyoma: available medical treatments and new possible therapeutic options. J Clin Endocrinol Metab. 2013;98:921-34.
12. De Leo V, Morgante G, La Marca A, Musacchio MC, Sorace M, Cavicchioli C, et al. A benefit-risk assessment of medical treatment for uterine leiomyomas. Drug Saf. 2002;25:759-79.
13. Lethaby A, Vollenhoven B, Sowter M. Pre-operative GnRH analogue therapy before hysterectomy or myomectomy for uterine fibroids. Cochrane Database Syst Rev. 2000:CD000547.
14. Palomba S, Affinito P, Di Carlo C, Bifulco G, Nappi C. Long-term administration of tibolone plus gonadotropin-releasing hormone agonist for the treatment of uterine leiomyomas: Effectiveness and effects on vasomotor symptoms, bone mass, and lipid profiles. Fertil Steril. 1999;72:889-95.
15. Palomba S, Orio F, Jr, Morelli M, Russo T, Pellicano M, Nappi C, et al. Raloxifene administration in women treated with gonadotropin-releasing hormone agonist for uterine leiomyomas: effects on bone metabolism. J Clin Endocrinol Metab. 2002; 87:4476-81.
16. Sabry M, Al-Hendy A. Innovative oral treatments of uterine leiomyoma. Obstet Gynecol Int. 2012;2012:943635.
17. Reissmann T, Diedrich K, Comaru-Schally AM, Schally AV. Introduction of LHRH-antagonists into the treatment of gynaecological disorders. Hum Reprod. 1994;9:769.
18. Kettel LM, Murphy AA, Morales AJ, Rivier J, Vale W, Yen SS. Rapid regression of uterine leiomyomas in response to daily administration of gonadotropin-releasing hormone antagonist. Fertil Steril. 1993; 60:642-6.
19. Chwalisz K, Perez MC, Demanno D, Winkel C, Schubert G, Elger W. Selective progesterone receptor modulator development and use in the treatment of leiomyomata and endometriosis. Endocr Rev. 2005;26:423-5.
20. Feng C, Meldrum S, Fiscella K. Improved quality of life is partly explained by fewer symptoms after treatment of fibroids with mifepristone. Int J Gynaecol Obstet. 2010; 109:121-4.
21. Kulshrestha V, Kriplani A, Agarwal N, Sareen N, Garg P, Hari S, et al. Low dose mifepristone in medical management of uterine leiomyoma – an experience from a tertiary care hospital from north India. Indian J Med Res. 2013;137:1154-62.
22. Shen Q, Hua Y, Jiang W, Zhang W, Chen M, Zhu X. Effects of mifepristone on uterine leiomyoma in premenopausal women: a meta-analysis. Fertil Steril. 2013;100:1722-6.
23. Murphy AA, Kettel LM, Morales AJ, Roberts VJ, Yen SS. Regression of uterine leiomyomata in response to the antiprogesterone RU 486. J Clin Endocrinol Metab. 1993;76:513-7.
24. Reinsch RC, Murphy AA, Morales AJ, Yen SS. The effects of RU 486 and leuprolide acetate on uterine artery blood flow in the fibroid uterus: a prospective, randomized study. Am J Obstet Gynecol. 1994;170:1623-7.
25. Donnez J, Tomaszewski J, Vázquez F, Bouchard P, Lemieszczuk B, Baró F, et al. Ulipristal acetate versus leuprolide acetate for uterine fibroids. N Engl J Med. 2012;366:421-32.
26. Donnez J, Donnez O, Matule D, Ahrendt HJ, Hudecek R, Zatik J, et al. Long-term medical management of uterine fibroids with ulipristal acetate. Fertil Steril. 2016;105:165-173.e4.
27. Deng L, Wu T, Chen XY, Xie L, Yang J. Selective estrogen receptor modulators (SERMs) for uterine leiomyomas. Cochrane Database Syst Rev. 2012;10:CD005287.
28. Lingxia X, Taixiang W, Xiaoyan C. Selective estrogen receptor modulators (SERMs) for uterine leiomyomas. Cochrane Database Syst Rev. 2007:CD005287.

29. Wu T, Chen X, Xie L. Selective estrogen receptor modulators (SERMs) for uterine leiomyomas. Cochrane Database Syst Rev. 2007;4:CD005287.
30. Ishikawa H, Reierstad S, Demura M, Rademaker AW, Kasai T, Inoue M, et al. High aromatase expression in uterine leiomyoma tissues of African-American women. J Clin Endocrinol Metab. 2009;94:1752-6.
31. Duhan N, Madaan S, Sen J. Role of the aromatase inhibitor letrozole in the management of uterine leiomyomas in premenopausal women. Eur J Obstet Gynecol Reprod Biol. 2013;171:329-32.
32. Hilário SG, Bozzini N, Borsari R, Baracat EC. Action of aromatase inhibitor for treatment of uterine leiomyoma in perimenopausal patients. Fertil Steril. 2009;91:240-3.
33. Brito LG, Candido-dos-Reis FJ, Magario FA, Sabino-de-Freitas MM. Effect of the aromatase inhibitor anastrozole on uterine and leiomyoma Doppler blood flow in patients scheduled for hysterectomy: a pilot study. Ultrasound Obstet Gynecol. 2012;40:119-20.

CHAPTER 19

Challenges in Cesarean Section with Fibroids

Upma Saxena

■ INTRODUCTION

Fibroid, myoma, and leiomyoma are synonymous terms for benign smooth muscle tumors arising from myometrium of the uterus. Fibroids represent the most common female benign tumors in reproductive age,[1] and they attain a large size during this period. Uterine fibroids complicate between 1.6% to 10.7% of pregnancies.[2] The prevalence of fibroids depends on whether the diagnosis is made in the first trimester versus the second trimester, the size threshold for reporting, and the demographic characteristics of the population. The prevalence of fibroids varies with race and increases with an increase in maternal age. In a prospective cohort study, including nearly 2,800 patients at 12 clinical sites in the United States, the prevalence of fibroids at any time during pregnancy was 12% and 32% in patients of 19–25 years and 35–42 years of age, respectively.[3]

■ EFFECTS OF PREGNANCY ON FIBROID

Changes in pregnancy hormones, especially estrogen and progesterone, uterine blood flow and beta-human chorionic gonadotropin (β-hCG) levels affect the volume of fibroid. In a prospective cohort study in the United States, change in total fibroid volume was found to be affected by the initial volume.[3] The trend of volume of fibroid that was observed was an increase in volume in patients with small volume at first visualization [diameter ≤1 cm; mean increase 2.0%; 95% confidence interval (CI) −0.3 to 4.5% per week], minimal or no change in patients with initial medium volume (diameter 1 to <3 cm; mean decrease 0.5%; 95% CI −2.0 to 1.0% per week), and decreasing trend in patients with initial large volumes (diameter ≥3 cm; mean decrease 2.2%; 95% CI −3.4 to −1.0% per week).[4]

Ninety percent of patients diagnosed with fibroid in the first trimester will show shrinkage of the fibroid, and only 10% will show increase in fibroid size when they are reevaluated 3–6 months postpartum.[5] Use of progestin-only contraception postnatally will hamper this postnatal regression.

In pregnant patients, fibroids typically do not show symptoms. However, if they do, it can be pain, pelvic pressure, or vaginal bleeding. Pain is the most commonly experienced symptom, and its frequency tends to increase with the size of the fibroid, particularly in cases of large fibroids, and it is due to degeneration and torsion.[6]

Fibroid-related pain typically arises during the late first or the early second trimester, coinciding with the period of the most significant fibroid growth. The rapid enlargement of fibroids can result in a relative reduction in blood flow, leading to ischemia and necrosis which is known as "red degeneration" and may be associated with the release of prostaglandins. Additionally, pedunculated fibroids may undergo torsion, which can cause acute exacerbation of pain.

EFFECTS OF FIBROID ON PREGNANCY

The location of the fibroid is a major determinant of the complications of pregnancy. Subserosal fibroids rarely lead to pregnancy complications; it is mostly submucosal or large intramural fibroids that affect the maternal or neonatal outcomes. Submucosal fibroids interfere with implantation, placentation, and ongoing pregnancy. During pregnancy, increased incidences of abortions, malpresentations, preterm birth, placenta previa, and placental abruption have been observed.[7-10] Fibroid arising from the cervix or occupying the whole of lower segment myoma can lead to obstructed labor in the intrapartum period, resulting in increased incidence of cesarean section or dysfunctional labor.[8] Postpartum complications can be retained placenta, subinvolution of the uterus, postpartum endomyometritis, and hemorrhage.[8] There are no clinical data suggesting that fibroids result in an increased risk of preterm prelabor rupture of membranes, fetal growth restriction, fetal demise, or preeclampsia.[8]

ROLE OF MYOMECTOMY IN PREGNANCY

The need for myomectomy during pregnancy should be individualized based on the location and size of the fibroid, the symptoms experienced by the patient, and past obstetric history. It has always been traditionally taught to avoid myomectomy during pregnancy, unless it is unavoidable, due to the increased risk of bleeding which may even require hysterectomy in order to achieve intraoperative hemostasis.

In a systematic review involving 97 patients, abdominal pain emerged as the most prevalent preoperative symptom, reported by 80% of the patients and serving as the primary indication for surgery. Fever was the second most common preoperative symptom, observed in 12% patients. The median gestational age of myomectomy was 16 weeks, with a range of 6–26 weeks. 75% of patients underwent removal of a single fibroid, while the remaining one quarter underwent myomectomy for multiple fibroids. The majority (73%) of myomectomies were performed for pedunculated fibroids, while in 39% of patients it was done for intramural fibroids.

The median estimated blood loss during surgery was 350 mL, and only five patients required transfusions. In five cases, pregnancy loss occurred postoperatively. The mean gestational ages at birth for patients undergoing single versus multiple myomectomies were 37.2 versus 36.8 weeks, with cesarean birth rates of 51% versus 83%. While most ongoing pregnancies proceeded without complications, one patient experienced full-thickness myometrial necrosis with abscess formation and exposure of the amniotic sac following the resection of a degenerating pedunculated leiomyoma using monopolar diathermy at 17 weeks' gestation. However, it was managed successfully with antibiotic therapy, incision and drainage of abscess, and repair of the defect. Elective cesarean section was performed for this patient at 37 completed weeks.[11]

In a meta-analysis primarily comprising retrospective studies involving patients undergoing myomectomy concurrently with cesarean section, the authors noted a significant decline in hemoglobin levels (mean difference of 0.25–0.27 mg/dL), along with an approximately 40% increase in blood transfusion rates and prolonged hospital stays.[12] However, the results of this study were not graded on the basis of the location and type of myomas, which significantly determine the risk of hemorrhage. Subserosal fibroids that are pedunculated tend to have the most favorable outcome.

EFFECT OF PRIOR MYOMECTOMY ON PREGNANCY

Women who had a pedunculated fibroid removed do not require special monitoring during pregnancy. Prior hysteroscopic removal of a submucosal fibroid may increase the risk of Asherman syndrome and placenta accreta spectrum. In patients with a history of prior myomectomy, an ultrasound examination should be performed in the late second or early third trimester to exclude placenta accreta spectrum. The extent and site of the previous uterine surgery determine the timing and mode of future delivery.

It is recommended to schedule an elective cesarean delivery between 36^{+0} and 37^{+0} weeks of gestation, before the onset of labor, for patients with a history of prior extensive or complicated myomectomy. In extensive myomectomy, there is deep encroachment of the myometrium by the fibroid needing its extensive dissection, for the removal of one or several intramural or submucosal fibroids of significant size, followed by extensive uterine reconstruction. Just opening of the uterine cavity does not qualify as an extensive myomectomy: however, there is no universally agreed-upon definition.

In cases of prior nonextensive, uncomplicated, intramyometrial myomectomy, a trial of labor can be carried out at as late as 38^{+6} weeks in a tertiary center equipped with facilities for continuous intrapartum fetal monitoring, ready access to obstetric anesthesia, and facility for emergency cesarean available round the clock. The risk of uterine rupture after myomectomy is almost similar to that during trial of labor after a previous cesarean section.[13]

MODE OF DELIVERY IN PREGNANCY WITH FIBROID

Most women with fibroids will have a successful vaginal birth and should be offered a trial of labor. Cesarean section is reserved for standard obstetric indications such as malpresentation and failure to progress.

Elective cesarean section may be considered in the following conditions:[14]
- Huge lower uterine segment or cervical fibroids which can lead to obstructed labor.
- Third-trimester ultrasonography finding suggestive of fibroid being located between the fetal head and the cervix.
- Women with prior extensive transmyometrial myomectomy.

CESAREAN SECTION IN PREGNANCY WITH FIBROID

There is an increased likelihood of cesarean birth (unadjusted odds ratio 3.7; 95% CI 3.5–3.9), particularly when the fibroid is situated in the lower uterine segment. This elevated cesarean birth rate is attributed to a higher risk of malpresentation, dysfunctional labor, obstructed labor, and an increased prevalence of abruption, due to implantation of placenta over the fibroid, causing abnormalities in the fetal heart rate.

During cesarean section, hysterotomy with a low transverse incision is preferred; however, when it is difficult to access the lower uterine segment, in case of a large lower segment fibroid, classical cesarean section may be needed for hysterotomy incisions.[15]

TIPS AND TRICKS FOR CLASSICAL CESAREAN SECTION

An infraumbilical midline vertical incision, 12–14 cm in length, should be made. An assistant should compress the uterus on each side of the wound toward the midline, during closure of the incision, to achieve good approximation. As classical incisions are thicker, they should be repaired in three layers to prevent dead space and later abscess formation, reducing febrile morbidity. The first layer should be closed with interrupted sutures, excluding the decidua, to avoid endometrial inversion, which leads to incomplete scar healing and endometriosis/adenomyosis later. The second layer should also be closed with interrupted sutures, and the serosal layer should be closed with continuous locking/figure-of-eight or Z suture/baseball sutures. After closure of the uterine incision, an adhesion barrier patch, such as Interceed or Seprafilm, should be applied.

OPERATIVE CONSIDERATIONS IN CESAREAN SECTION WITH FIBROID

Whenever preparing a pregnant patient with fibroid for cesarean section, one should be prepared for intrapartum or postpartum hemorrhage (PPH), especially in patients with placenta implanted over large fibroid or lower uterine segment occupied by a huge fibroid anteriorly. So adequate blood products should be arranged. The patient and her relatives should be counselled' for the same and obtain consent for cesarean hysterectomy/myomectomy.

Preoperative bilateral iliac artery balloon catheters should be inserted. Ultrasound should be performed either before or during labor to map the location of large uterine fibroids. This aids in deciding the placement of optimal hysterotomy incision at the time of cesarean section. Transection of the fibroid capsule during hysterotomy must be avoided as its breach will make closure of the incision feasible only after performing intraoperative myomectomy. Even a peripartum hysterectomy may be needed after myomectomy to achieve hemostasis, if hysterotomy closure is not attained.

Injection tranexamic acid, oxytocin, compression of uterine artery by tourniquet, ligation of uterine artery at its origin, and intramyometrium injection of vasopressin or tablet misoprostol can be used intraoperatively to control hemorrhage.[16]

INDICATIONS FOR CESAREAN MYOMECTOMY IN THE PAST

Cesarean intramyometrial myomectomy was generally avoided for fibroid >6 cm because of the risk of severe hemorrhage as uterus at term receives about 17% of the total cardiac output.

Earlier cesarean myomectomy was done *only* when:
- Symptomatic pedunculated fibroids and small fibroid
- To prevent necrobiosis in the postpartum period
- Fibroid causing pain
- Atypical looking fibroid intraoperative
- Tertiary center with availability of blood products
- Transection of capsule of fibroid during hysterotomy
- Surgeon has appropriate expertise.

DISADVANTAGES OF CESAREAN MYOMECTOMY

Massive intraoperative bleeding during cesarean section is the deadliest complication of myomectomy. Removal of a large fibroid during cesarean section leads to a higher rate of uterine rupture during pregnancy at a later date. Hence, it was commonly recommended that myomectomies be avoided as much as possible during cesarean delivery.

ADVANTAGES OF CESAREAN MYOMECTOMY

Performing cesarean myomectomy in resource-limited settings can offer significant benefits:
- It can prevent the additional morbidity associated with a repeat procedure, such as laparotomy for fibroid removal, and the need for subsequent anesthesia.
- Cesarean myomectomy has cost benefits as it may prevent many complications of fibroids in future pregnancy, that is, PPH, myoma degeneration, abortion, preterm birth, twisting of subserosal fibroid with pedicle, or "red" degeneration.
- It could potentially reduce subinvolution of puerperal uterus and other fibroid-induced problems such as menorrhagia, anemia, and pain.
- In comparison to nongravid uterus, the size of fibroids to the uterus is relatively decreased during pregnancy, leading to a smaller incision on the uterus, at the time of myomectomy being performed during cesarean section.
- During pregnancy, elasticity of myometrium increases and fragility decreases, so its suturing becomes easier during cesarean section.
- "Classical" incision should be used while performing cesarean myomectomy for large fibroids occupying whole of the lower uterine segment.

In a retrospective cohort study, pregnant women with uterine fibroids having myomectomy performed during cesarean section (study group; $n = 91$) were compared with those who did not have myomectomy (control group; $n = 87$). There were insignificant differences in the amount of blood transfusion and postoperative hemoglobin levels between the two groups. However, the operative time was significantly increased in the study group undergoing myomectomy compared to the control group ($p < 0.001$). Postoperative hospital stay was also, significantly higher in the myomectomy group ($p < 0.001$). The authors concluded that myomectomy can be safely performed during cesarean section, with the added benefits of preventing repeat operation to remove fibroids at a later date which outweigh the prolonged operating time and longer hospital stay.[17]

A prospective study was conducted at a tertiary care referral center, which included 34 pregnant women in whom myomectomy was performed during elective or emergency cesarean section. The authors analyzed factors such as age, parity, type of myomas, intraoperative and postoperative morbidity, time taken for surgery, and hospital stay duration. They found no significant difference in mean hemoglobin levels preoperatively and postoperatively. Additionally, no patients experienced PPH requiring cesarean hysterectomy, and only two patients required postoperative blood transfusion. The mean duration of surgery was 58.4 ± 8.94 minutes and the mean hospital stay was 6.7 ± 1.6 days. The authors concluded that with advancements in anesthesia techniques and blood transfusion capabilities, cesarean myomectomy can be performed safely by senior obstetricians in judiciously selected patients.[18]

A study was carried out in Taiwan in which the authors found that myomectomy during cesarean birth in patients with uterine fibroids was safe and had good outcome. The literature was reviewed and the outcomes of 17 studies involving 542 patients who underwent simultaneous myomectomy and cesarean section were analyzed. The authors found that performing myomectomy during cesarean section was feasible and safe, with low rates of complications such as bleeding, infection, and wound dehiscence. Simultaneous myomectomy did not increase the risk of adverse obstetric outcomes such as preterm birth, PPH, or uterine rupture. Also, the authors recommended that the decision to perform myomectomy during cesarean section should be individualized and based on factors such as the size, location, and number of fibroids, as well as the patient's age and desire for future fertility. They emphasized that only senior obstetricians should perform myomectomy simultaneously during cesarean, and patients should receive adequate counseling about the potential risks and benefits of the procedure. The authors concluded that this approach may lead to lower rates of repeat cesarean and future fertility preservation.[19]

In a systematic review and meta-analysis encompassing 17 studies involving 6,545 women, the outcomes investigated included hemorrhage, mean change in hemoglobin, operative time, need for blood transfusion, febrile morbidity, and hospital stay. The review comprised 4,702 (71.85%) patients in the cesarean myomectomy group and 1,843 (28.15%) patients in the cesarean section group.

Statistically significant but clinically insignificant decreases in hemoglobin levels were observed in the cesarean myomectomy group compared to cesarean section alone (MD = 0.27; 95% CI = 0.08–0.45; p = 0.005; very low quality). The cesarean myomectomy group exhibited a significantly higher need for blood transfusion compared to cesarean section alone [relative risk (RR) = 1.45; 95% CI = 1.05–1.99; p = 0.02; high quality]. There was no significant difference in the incidence of hemorrhage (RR = 1.16; 95% CI = 0.86–1.56; p = 0.32; moderate quality) or fever (RR = 1.17; 95% CI = 0.83–1.65; p = 0.36; moderate quality) between the two groups. The meta-analysis suggested that cesarean myomectomy was associated with a clinically insignificant increase in operative time, blood loss, and hospital stay, particularly in cases involving multiple and large-sized myomas. The authors suggested that cesarean myomectomy is preferable over cesarean section alone, when myomectomy is carried out by an experienced obstetrician using effective hemostatic techniques at referral centers.[12]

■ CONCLUSION

Women with fibroids can have a successful vaginal birth after trial of labor. Elective cesarean for fibroids should be performed only when there is huge fibroid occupying the lower segment or replacing the cervix. Ultrasound mapping of fibroid in the gravid uterus should be done preoperatively or intraoperatively to avoid inadvertently transecting capsule of fibroid. Classical incisions are needed for large lower segment fibroid, and it should be repaired in three layers. Preoperative counseling of women should be done about risks and benefits of myomectomy. The decision to perform myomectomy during cesarean should be individualized. With the availability of safe anesthesia and blood transfusion facilities, cesarean myomectomy is a cost-effective and patient-friendly surgical procedure when performed by senior obstetricians at a tertiary-level hospital.

REFERENCES

1. Sparic R, Mirkovic L, Malvasi A, Tinelli A. Epidemiology of uterine myomas: a review. Inte J Fertil Steril. 2016;9:424-35.
2. Stout MJ, Odibo AO, Graseck AS, Macones GA, Crane JP, Cahill AG. Leiomyomas at routine second-trimester ultrasound examination and adverse obstetric outcomes. Obstet Gynecol. 2010;116:1056.
3. Mitro SD, Peddada S, Chen Z, Buck Louis GM, Gleason JL, Zhang C, et al. Natural history of fibroids in pregnancy: National Institute of Child Health and Human Development Fetal Growth Studies - Singletons cohort. Fertil Steril. 2022;118:656.
4. Coutinho LM, Assis WA, Spagnuolo-Souza A, Reis FM. Uterine fibroids and pregnancy: how do they affect each other? Reprod Sci. 2022;29(8):2145-51.
5. Laughlin SK, Hartmann KE, Baird DD. Postpartum factors and natural fibroid regression. Am J Obstet Gynecol. 2011;204:496.e1.
6. Lam SJ, Best S, Kumar S. The impact of fibroid characteristics on pregnancy outcome. Am J Obstet Gynecol. 2014;211:395.e1.
7. Gabbe SG, Niebyl JR, Simpson JL. Obstetrics: Normal and Problem Pregnancies, 4th edition. Pennsylvania: Churchill Livingstone; 2008. p. 739.
8. Klatsky PC, Tran ND, Caughey AB, Fujimoto VY. Fibroids and reproductive outcomes: a systematic literature review from conception to delivery. Am J Obstet Gynecol. 2008;198:357.
9. Jenabi E, Ebrahimzadeh Zagami S. The association between uterine leiomyoma and placenta abruption: a meta-analysis. J Matern Fetal Neonatal Med. 2017;30:2742.
10. Jenabi E, Fereidooni B. The uterine leiomyoma and placenta previa: a meta-analysis. J Matern Fetal Neonatal Med. 2019;32:1200.
11. Spyropoulou K, Kosmas I, Tsakiridis I, Mamopoulos A, Kalogiannidis I, Athanasiadis A, et al. Myomectomy during pregnancy: a systematic review. Eur J Obstet Gynecol Reprod Biol. 2020;254:15.
12. Goyal M, Dawood AS, Elbohoty SB, Abbas AM, Singh P, Melana N, et al. Cesarean myomectomy in the last ten years; A true shift from contraindication to indication: a systematic review and meta-analysis. Eur J Obstet Gynecol Reprod Biol. 2021;256:145.
13. Gambacorti-Passerini Z, Gimovsky AC, Locatelli A, Berghella V. Trial of labor after myomectomy and uterine rupture: a systematic review. Acta Obstet Gynecol Scand. 2016;95:724.
14. Tian J, Hu W. Cervical leiomyomas in pregnancy: report of 17 cases. Aust N Z J Obstet Gynaecol. 2012;52:258.
15. Kan A. Classical cesarean section. Surg J (N Y). 2020;6(Suppl. 2):S98-103.
16. Abdul IF, Amadu MB, Adesina KT, Olarinoye AO, Omokanye LO. Adjunctive use of tranexamic acid to tourniquet in reducing haemorrhage during abdominal myomectomy – a randomized controlled trial. Eur J Obstet Gynecol Reprod Biol. 2019;242:150-58.
17. El-Refaie W, Hassan M, Abdelhafez MS. Myomectomy during cesarean section: a retrospective cohort study. J Gynecol Obstet Hum Reprod. 2020:101900.
18. Bala R, Kamal P, Nagpal M, Singh S. Current status of cesarean section myomectomy-prospective ongoing study. Int J Reprod Contracept Obstet Gynecol. 2019;8(8):3189.
19. Liu CH, Chang WH, Yeh CC, Wang PH. Simultaneous myomectomy during cesarean section. Taiwan J Obstet Gynecol. 2021;60(3):397-8.

CHAPTER 20

Uterine Smooth Muscle Tumors of Uncertain Malignant Potential

Deepali Raina

■ INTRODUCTION

The spectrum of uterine smooth muscle tumors has a typical benign leiomyoma at one end and a malignant leiomyosarcoma (LMS) at the other end. Uterine smooth muscle tumor of uncertain malignant potential (STUMP) is a subtype of uterine smooth muscle tumor lying somewhere between the two extremes. The World Health Organization (WHO) classification defines a STUMP as a uterine smooth muscle tumor that cannot be diagnosed unequivocally as benign or malignant.[1] Most of the literature on uterine STUMP are in the form of case reports and case series. Excessive menstrual bleeding, heaviness in abdomen, a palpable mass in lower abdomen, and anemia are the usual presenting symptoms though many patients are asymptomatic as well. In most of the patients, the diagnosis is made postoperatively on the basis of the final histopathology report as it is difficult to distinguish STUMP from benign leiomyomas and LMS based on symptoms, clinical examination, or radiology. The median age at diagnosis is 40–45 years. The rate of recurrence varies from 7 to 36.4% and the 5-year overall survival rate of patients is over 90%.[2]

■ PATHOLOGY

An established diagnostic criterion for uterine STUMP is not available. They resemble fibroids both grossly and microscopically. These tumors have a well-circumscribed and nonencapsulated appearance. The cut surface is white with a whorled appearance and occasional areas of infarction, hemorrhage, and myxoid change. The median size is 6–8 cm.[3] Histopathologic diagnosis of STUMP is based on the features of cellular atypia, tumor cell necrosis, and mitotic index.[4] Genetically, STUMP is a heterogenous group of tumors with genomic profiles that can harbor small or rare chromosomal alterations to high chromosomal instability. However, the chromosomal alterations are low when compared to LMS. These genetic alterations can be measured with the help of newer techniques like array-comparative genomic hybridization analysis, etc.[5]

Many immunohistochemical markers are helpful in differentiating ambiguous tumors that are difficult to diagnose and in providing prognostic information. Progesterone receptor and estrogen receptor expression are frequently present in STUMP and leiomyomas but occur much less frequently in LMS. The levels of Ki-67, a cell proliferation marker, are high in LMS, but significantly less in STUMP and fibroids. P16 is expressed in 76.4% of LMSs, 38.4% of STUMPs, and 10.3% of benign leiomyomas. P53 is strongly expressed in LMS but only weakly positive or negative expression in STUMP and other benign soft-tissue tumors and leiomyomas.

STUMP also stain positive for desmin, H-caldesmon, smooth muscle actin, and Wilms tumor (WT) 1 while being cluster of differentiation (CD) 10 negative.[6] None of these immunohistochemistry (IHC) markers are exclusive and there is a significant overlap in expression of these markers across the smooth muscle tumor spectrum. Thus, histopathology and IHC markers along with genomic profiling go hand in hand for the characterization of STUMP tumors.

CLINICAL FEATURES AND DIAGNOSIS

It is close to impossible to differentiate STUMP from other smooth muscle tumors preoperatively. Symptoms are similar to those of leiomyomas like vague pelvic discomfort, dysmenorrhea, abnormal uterine bleeding, anemia, infertility, and dysuria. Over 80% of the patients are premenopausal. Almost all of the tumors are uterus confined and metastasis is not a primary presenting feature, though extremely rare cases of STUMP with pulmonary metastasis are reported.[7] No clear risk factors have been identified.

At present, magnetic resonance imaging (MRI) can only be used to differentiate STUMP and LMS from benign leiomyomas. MRI parameters that raise the suspicion of uterine soft-tissue tumors not being benign are necrosis, irregular margins, endometrial infiltration, heterogeneous architecture, and increased diffusion restriction, but their positive predictive value in diagnosing STUMP or LMS is low. Sarcomas and STUMPs are also usually larger than leiomyomas and have higher signal intensity on T2-weighted images. Like MRI, there are no specific ultrasound characteristics for STUMP as well. However, features like increased vascularization with high Doppler enhancement, irregular outline, and necrotic areas do point toward possible malignancy. The usefulness of PET-CT scan is limited too in differential diagnosis. The STUMPs and LMSs may show a typical "hollow ball sign", a feature which is absent in leiomyomas. However, this sign is created by the areas of coagulative tumor necrosis which may be seen in many other situations as well and is therefore not pathognomonic for STUMPs.[8] For all practical purposes, the aim of imaging is to differentiate between a benign fibroid and a potential malignant or STUMP tumor so that care can be taken while operating to avoid morcellation and prefer intact removal of the soft-tissue tumor.

MANAGEMENT AND FOLLOW-UP

The diagnosis of STUMP is typically made by postoperative histopathological examination. For patients who have completed their family or have no desire to get pregnant, total hysterectomy with or without bilateral salpingo-oophorectomy is the treatment of choice.[8] The overall rate of STUMP recurrence after hysterectomy is variably mentioned in the literature. The sites of recurrence are unpredictable too and it is thought that almost two-thirds may have a distant recurrence in lungs, liver, peritoneum, or bones. In many retrospective analyses, the rate of recurrence after myomectomy alone has been seen to be around 6%. Therefore, for patients who are of reproductive age and desire fertility, myomectomy may be a feasible option too.[9] In conservative surgical management, one-third of the recurrences will be in the uterus itself. Adjuvant hormone therapy or chemotherapy is of no proven value in the management of STUMP. Genomic analysis may be a good predictor of recurrence and can be used for selecting high-risk patients to offer more intense follow-up. Studies about the role of morcellation for

STUMPs are limited. Morcellation without the use of an endobag is associated with an almost three times higher tumor recurrence rate in STUMP compared to intact tumor excision or morcellation within an endobag and should never be done.[8] A detailed discussion about the possible risks should be done with the patients and an informed consent must be obtained before surgery for protected morcellation if intended.

Most STUMP relapses occur after 5 years of diagnosis. STUMP with significant atypia alone or tumor cell necrosis alone exhibits average risks of recurrence of 17–18%, while the recurrence rate for tumors with a high mitotic index alone is not very high.[3] The recurrences may be in the form of STUMP or even LMS. Patients should be under close follow-up considering the unpredictable behavior of the disease.[7] A follow-up interval of 6 months for the first 5 years and then yearly surveillance for a period of 5 more years is recommended. Follow-up should include annual chest radiography and contrast-enhanced MRI of abdomen and pelvis.[10]

Surgery is the most beneficial treatment for relapsed cases, though radiation therapy and cisplatin and doxorubicin-based chemotherapy have been tried as well. Hormonal therapy with progesterone, aromatase inhibitors, or gonadotropin-releasing hormone analogs may be prescribed as well.[11] None of these modalities has been proven to be effective in any randomized controlled study, and treatment should be individualized.

CONCLUSION

Uterine STUMP present a diagnostic challenge due to their intermediate nature between benign leiomyomas and malignant LMSs. With no universally recognized diagnostic criteria, a combination of histopathological examination, immunohistochemical markers, and genomic profiling is essential for accurate diagnosis and management. Treatment typically involves surgical resection, with total hysterectomy recommended for patients who have completed childbearing. Close follow-up is crucial due to the unpredictable behavior of STUMP. Further research is needed to establish more definitive guidelines for the diagnosis and management of this complex and rare entity.

REFERENCES

1. Oliva E, Carcangiu ML, Carinelli SG. Tumours of the uterine corpus: mesenchymal tumours: smooth muscle tumour of uncertain malignant potential. In: Kurman RJ, Carcangiu ML, Herrington CS, Young RH (Eds). World Health Organization Classification of Tumors of Female Reproductive Organs. Lyon: IARC Press; 2014. pp. 138-9.
2. Liu HT, Wong CN, Wong CN, Liu FS. Uterine smooth muscle tumor of uncertain malignant potential: A review of current knowledge. Taiwan J Obstet Gynecol. 2022;61(6):935-40.
3. Di Giuseppe J, Grelloni C, Giuliani L, Delli Carpini G, Giannella L, Ciavattini A. Recurrence of Uterine Smooth Muscle Tumor of Uncertain Malignant Potential: a Systematic Review of the Literature. Cancers (Basel). 2022;14(9):2323.
4. Gupta M, Laury AL, Nucci MR, Quade BJ. Predictors of adverse outcome in uterine smooth muscle tumours of uncertain malignant potential (STUMP): a clinicopathological analysis of 22 cases with a proposal for the inclusion of additional histological parameters. Histopathology. 2018;73:284-98.
5. Croce S, Ducoulombier A, Ribeiro A, Lesluyes T, Noel JC, Amant F, et al. Genome profiling is an efficient tool to avoid the STUMP classification of uterine smooth muscle lesions: a comprehensive array-genomic hybridization analysis of 77 tumors. Mod Pathol. 2018;31(5):816-28.
6. Zheng YY, Liu XB, Mao YY, Lin MH. Smooth muscle tumor of uncertain malignant potential (STUMP): a clinicopathologic

analysis of 26 cases. Int J Clin Exp Pathol. 2020;13(4):818-26.
7. Kotsopoulos IC, Barbetakis N, Asteriou C, Voutsas MG. Uterine smooth muscle tumor of uncertain malignant potential: a rare cause of multiple pulmonary nodules. Indian J Med Paediatr Oncol. 2012;33(3):176-8.
8. Tinelli A, D'Oria O, Civino E, Morciano A, Hashmi AA, Baldini GM, et al. Smooth muscle tumor of uncertain malignant potential (STUMP): a comprehensive multidisciplinary update. Medicina (Kaunas). 2023; 59(8):1371.
9. Richtarova A, Boudova B, Dundr P, Lisa Z, Hlinecka K, Zizka Z, et al. Uterine smooth muscle tumors with uncertain malignant potential: analysis following fertility-saving procedures. Int J Gynecol Cancer. 2023; 33(5):701-6.
10. Bacanakgil BH, Deveci M, Karabuk E, Soyman Z. Uterine smooth muscle tumor of uncertain malignant potential: clinicopathologic-sonographic characteristics, follow-up and recurrence. World J Oncol. 2017;8(3):76-80.
11. Guntupalli SR, Ramirez PT, Anderson ML, Milam MR, Bodurka DC, Malpica A. Uterine smooth muscle tumor of uncertain malignant potential: a retrospective analysis. Gynecol Oncol. 2009;113(3):324-6.

CHAPTER 21

Atypical Leiomyoma

Ruchika Garg, Mousumi Das Ghosh

■ INTRODUCTION

Atypical leiomyomas (ALMs), also called pleomorphic leiomyomas, have distinct heterogeneous, histologic, and molecular features and may be a precursor lesion of leiomyosarcoma (LMS).[1] Existing literature is scarce as these are rare.

These uterine smooth muscle tumors have been categorized pathologically as six major types: (1) Leiomyoma (LM), (2) mitotically active leiomyoma, (3) cellular leiomyoma, (4) ALM, (5) smooth muscle tumor of uncertain malignant potential, (6) and LMS.[1] The triad of moderate to severe cytologic atypia, less than 10 mitoses per 10 high-power fields (HPF), and no coagulative tumor necrosis on histopathology defines them. LMS has tumor cell necrosis and mitotic counts >10/10 HPF.

■ DIAGNOSIS

Clinical features resemble those of ordinary LM like abnormal uterine bleeding, pelvic mass, pelvic pain, and anemia.[2] No specific risk factors have been associated with the diagnosis. The incidence is high in large-sized myomas, especially in women in their forties. Usually, the diagnosis is made postoperatively based on the histopathology report.

There are no precise imaging tests to diagnose before surgery. The gold standard for diagnosis is histopathology.[3] Magnetic resonance imaging (MRI) studies[4] may show a solid mass, cystic portion, and low signal on T2-weighted imaging. The tumors have benign behavior.[5] ALMs are rare in postmenopausal women.

■ MANAGEMENT

Suspicious uterine masses on preoperative imaging should have surgical management with histopathology diagnosis. Hence, myomectomy or hysterectomy is better than medical management or uterine fibroid embolization.[3] Also, power morcellation is better avoided if preoperative imaging studies suggest a LM variant. Hysterectomy is the treatment of choice for ALM and myomectomy may be an option for fertility-sparing cases.

■ HISTOPATHOLOGY

The new World Health Organization (WHO) Classification of Tumors of Female Reproductive Organs has renamed this variant as leiomyoma with bizarre nuclei (LM-BN). When the atypia is at most multifocal and the neoplasm has been completely sampled, it is termed "ALM with minimal, if any, recurrence potential".[6]

■ TYPES

Atypical leiomyoma is classified into type I and type II, based primarily on nuclear features[7] and architectural differences. The two subtypes also differ when immunohistochemical (IHC) and molecular patterns are compared. Type II tumors have higher rates of immunoreactivity for p16, p53, and HMGA2 and showed *MED12* mutations than the type I counterparts. Type I tumors may be related to fumarate hydratase mutations, while type II ALM appear to arise in a background of usual-type LMs.

The diagnosis of ALMs, smooth muscle tumors of uncertain malignant potential (STUMPs), and LMSs is confusing, so p16, p21, PR, bcl-2, p53, and Ki-67 expression should be looked for.[5]

■ PROGNOSIS

Prognosis is generally good with extrauterine and intra-abdominal recurrence rate of <2% and low risk of distant metastasis.[3] Follow-up without adjuvant therapy is recommended.

LEIOMYOSARCOMA

Uterine sarcomas can be divided into three categories:[8]
1. Uterine LMS (uLMS; anomalous proliferation of the myometrial layer of the uterus)
2. Endometrial stromal sarcoma (anomalous proliferation of the connective tissue underlining the endometrium)
3. Undifferentiated sarcoma.

Uterine sarcomas are rare malignant tumors of mesenchymal origin, representing 3–7% of primary malignant uterine tumors with an incidence of 0.7 per 100,000 women.[4,9] Globally, the average age at diagnosis is 55 years. It has a poor prognosis, with a 5-year survival rate of 17–55%, even when it is discovered at an early stage. The estimated prevalence of occult LMS is 0.12 per 1,000 surgeries.[10]

■ ETIOLOGY[11]

Definite etiology for LMS is not identified. LMS might be a de novo entity. Prior history of radiotherapy or Tamoxifen intake is a risk factor for the development of LMS. Patients with genetic syndromes like hereditary retinoblastoma (*RB1* gene deletion) and Li–Fraumeni syndrome (mutation in the *TP53* gene) can develop LMS.

■ DIAGNOSIS

The preoperative detection of LMS is difficult due to the clinical similarity to ordinary LMs. There are no specific features in diagnosis. The most common presentation is mass effect from a growing lesion or abnormal uterine bleeding. Though ultrasound is used as first-line assessment, it cannot differentiate between benign and malignant tumors.[12]

Endometrial biopsy helps in diagnosis; however, a negative biopsy does not rule out LMS. Hysteroscopy with endometrial sampling improved preoperative detection of LMS by three-fold.[13] LM growing beyond menopause should undergo biopsy.[14]

CT scan or MRI can aid in staging. It is important to look for lung or liver metastasis as spread is mainly via the hematogenous route. LMSs usually present as solitary, heterogeneous, and poorly demarcated masses[15] with hemorrhage or necrosis. On MRI, enlarged lymph nodes, peritoneal implants, and a high diffusion-weighted MRI signal greater than that in endometrium may enable identification of LMS.[4] Positron emission tomography/computed tomography (PET/CT) remains limited because ordinary LMs can uptake 18F-fluorodeoxyglucose in PET/CT.[12]

■ HISTOPATHOLOGY

Marked nuclear atypia, high mitotic rate, tumor cell necrosis, and mitotic index are important factors in the diagnosis of uLMS. Histologically, spindle cell and nonspindle cell morphologies, and nonspindle type may have worse outcome.[12]

Immunohistochemical stains like desmin, smooth-muscle actin, and h-caldesmon confirm smooth-muscle origin, whereas histone deacetylase-8 and myocardin point to epithelioid tumors.

Immunopositivity for p16 and p53 with a high Ki-67 proliferation index helps differentiate benign from malignant tumors. LMS has a lower expression of estrogen (40% in LMS vs. 70% in LM) and progesterone receptors (38% in LMS vs. 88% in LM).

MANAGEMENT

It is best treated in centers experienced in treating sarcoma patients. Cases should be discussed in tumor board. Two staging systems are used for uterine sarcomas, including the 2018 Federation International Gynaecology and Obstetrics (FIGO) and the 2010 American Joint Committee on Cancer tumor, lymph node, and metastasis systems. The FIGO staging is more frequently applied in clinical practice.

FIGO STAGING FOR UTERINE SARCOMAS (2018)

- *Stage I:* Tumor limited to the uterus
  - *IA:* <5 cm in greatest dimension
  - *IB:* >5 cm in greatest dimension
- *Stage II:* Tumor extends beyond the uterus, within the pelvis
  - *IIA:* Adnexal involvement
  - *IIB:* Involvement of other pelvic tissues
- *Stage III:* Tumor infiltrates abdominal tissues (lesions must not just protrude into abdominal cavity)
  - *IIIA:* Tumor infiltrates abdominal tissues in one site
  - *IIIB:* Tumor infiltrates abdominal tissues in more than one site
  - *IIIC:* Involves pelvic and/or para-aortic lymph nodes
- *Stage IV:* Tumor invades pelvic organs and/or distant metastasis
  - *IVA:* Invasion of bladder or rectum
  - *IVB:* Distant metastases.

The goal of treatment is to control the symptoms, decrease tumor bulk, and prolong survival.[11] The treatment of choice is hysterectomy en bloc to avoid intraoperative rupture, morcellation, or spillage of tumor into the peritoneal cavity.[16] The decision regarding removal of adnexa is optional and the ovaries can be preserved if the tumor is limited to the uterus in young females.[17] However, most cases are diagnosed postoperatively based on the histopathology report and potential tumor spillage may upgrade the disease worsening the prognosis.

The role of retroperitoneal lymph node dissection is also debatable. As the incidence of metastases is low, pelvic and para-aortic lymph node dissection in routine practice may be avoided. However, lymphadenectomy can be performed as part of a cytoreduction in symptomatic patients with extensively advanced tumors. If optimal cytoreduction is done, adjuvant radiotherapy is not recommended in LMS. It may be considered in advanced stage, incompletely resected, or metastatic disease.

The role of chemotherapy with complete resection for uterus-limited disease is also controversial. Drugs used are doxorubicin, doxorubicin plus ifosfamide, gemcitabine, and gemcitabine plus docetaxel. The second-line therapy includes pazopanib, trabectedin, dacarbazine, or temozolomide or fixed dose-rate gemcitabine plus docetaxel after doxorubicin-treated failure. LMS has unbalanced karyotypes, severe genomic instability, and multiple genetic aberrations. As a result, LMS is considered moderately sensitive to chemotherapy. Efficacy studies of immunotherapy in uterine sarcomas are ongoing.[18]

PROGNOSIS

Leiomyosarcoma is an aggressive malignancy with late diagnosis. The most important prognostic factors are histologic grade, tumor size, tumor depth, age, disease stage, surgical margins, cellular atypia, mitotic rate, involvement of lymphovascular channels, lymph node positivity, oophorectomy, and presence or absence of necrosis.

CONCLUSION

A multidisciplinary team of gynecologists, pathologists, and oncologists is needed. Immunohistochemistry is recommended to investigate the overexpression of p16 and p53 to identify the cohort of patients at an increased risk of recurrence who may benefit from more aggressive surgical–oncological strategies.[6]

The standard treatment for uLMS is hysterectomy and complete cytoreduction of the tumor en bloc with adherent structures, even if not overtly infiltrated. Immunohistochemistry can help identify patients at higher risk of recurrence, guiding the implementation of more aggressive treatment strategies. Outcomes can be challenging, especially in advanced or recurrent cases. Treatment outcomes are disappointing, especially in patients with inoperable, locally advanced, recurrent, and/or metastatic diseases.

Artificial intelligence and MRI-based algorithms for assessing atypical uterine masses in routine clinical practice and diffusion-weighted imaging may help in future.[19]

REFERENCES

1. Singh S, Naik M, Behera JC, Mishra P. Atypical leiomyoma of the uterus: a case report. Int J Case Rep Images. 2015;7(1):55-9.
2. Rizzo A, Ricci AD, Saponara M, DE Leo A, Perrone AM, DE Iaco P, et al. Recurrent uterine smooth-muscle tumors of uncertain malignant potential (STUMP): State of The Art. Anticancer Res. 2020;40(3):1229-38.
3. Yun Sook K, Hyun Joo L. A case report of atypical uterine leiomyoma. Med Case Rep Study Protoc. 2021;2(11):e0168.
4. Abdel Wahab C, Jannot AS, Bonaffini PA, Bourillon C, Cornou C, Lefrère-Belda MA, et al. Diagnostic algorithm to differentiate benign atypical leiomyomas from malignant uterine sarcomas with diffusion-weighted MRI. Radiology. 2020;297(2):361-71.
5. Manxhuka-Kerliu S, Kerliu-Saliu I, Sahatciu-Meka V, Kerliu L, Shahini L. Atypical uterine leiomyoma: a case report and review of the literature. J Med Case Reports. 2016;10:22.
6. Dall'Asta A, Gizzo S, Musarò A, Quaranta M, Noventa M, Migliavacca C, et al. Uterine smooth muscle tumors of uncertain malignant potential (STUMP): Pathology, follow-up and recurrence. Int J Clin Exp Pathol. 2014;7(11):8136-42.
7. Ubago JM, Zhang Q, Kim JJ, Kong B, Wei JJ. Two subtypes of atypical leiomyoma: clinical, histologic, and molecular analysis. Am J Surg Pathol. 2016;40(7):923-33.
8. Surace A, Baù MG, Privitera S, Botta G, Danese S, Plazzotta C. Risk of unexpected uterine leiomyosarcoma during laparoscopic procedures: experience from a single tertiary institute in Italy. Int J Gynaecol Obstet. 2022;156(2):236-9.
9. Kalogiannidis I, Stavrakis T, Dagklis T, Petousis S, Nikolaidou C, Venizelos I, et al. A clinicopathological study of atypical leiomyomas: benign variant leiomyoma or smooth-muscle tumor of uncertain malignant potential. Oncol Lett. 2016;11(2):1425-28.
10. Pritts EA, Vanness DJ, Berek JS, Parker W, Feinberg R, Feinberg J, et al. The prevalence of occult leiomyosarcoma at surgery for

presumed uterine fibroids: a meta-analysis. Gynecol Surg. 2015;12(3):165-77.
11. Mangla A, Yadav U, Menon G. Leiomyosarcoma. In: StatPearls. Treasure Island (FL): StatPearls Publishing; 2024. Available from https://www.ncbi.nlm.nih.gov/books/NBK551667 [Last accessed June, 2024].
12. Horng HC, Wen KC, Wang PH, Chen YJ, Yen MS, Ng HT. Taiwan Association of Gynecology Systematic Review Group. Uterine sarcoma Part II-Uterine endometrial stromal sarcoma: The TAG systematic review. Taiwan J Obstet Gynecol. 2016;55(4):472-9.
13. Kho RM, Desai VB, Schwartz PE, Wright JD, Gross CP, Hutchison LM, et al. Endometrial sampling for preoperative diagnosis of uterine leiomyosarcoma. J Minim Invasive Gynecol. 2022;29(1):119-27.
14. Juhasz-Böss I, Gabriel L, Bohle RM, Horn LC, Solomayer EF, Breitbach GP. Uterine leiomyosarcoma. Oncol Res Treat. 2018;41(11):680-6.
15. Sun S, Bonaffini PA, Nougaret S, Fournier L, Dohan A, Chong J, et al. How to differentiate uterine leiomyosarcoma from leiomyoma with imaging. Diagn Interv Imaging. 2019;100(10):619-34.
16. George S, Serrano C, Hensley ML, Ray-Coquard I. Soft tissue and uterine leiomyosarcoma. J Clin Oncol. 2018;10;36(2):144-50.
17. Dunphy L, Sheridan G. Uterine leiomyosarcoma: a rare clinical entity. BMJ Case Rep. 2021;14(8):e244233.
18. Desar IME, Ottevanger PB, Benson C, van der Graaf WTA. Systemic treatment in adult uterine sarcomas. Crit Rev Oncol Hematol. 2018;122:10-20.
19. Méndez RJ. MRI to differentiate atypical leiomyoma from uterine sarcoma. Radiology. 2020;297(2):372-3.

Index

Page numbers followed by *f* refer to figure, and *t* refer to table.

A

Abdominal
  cavity 105
  closure 77
  hysterectomy 99
  incisions 73
  myomectomy 37, 72, 99
  surgery 92
Abruption, prevalence of 125
Acupuncture 16
Adenomyoma 31
Adenomyosis 31, 36*f*, 53, 117
Adhesion 77
  formation, preventing 69*f*
  prevention 77
Adnexa 89*f*
Adnexal pathologies 31
Amenorrhea 52, 53, 57
American Association of
    Gynecologic
    Laparoscopists 106
American College of
    Obstetricians and
    Gynecologists 67, 73
American Joint Committee on
    Cancer Tumor 136
Anastrazole 56, 58, 116
Anemia 98
Anesthesia 73, 80
Anomalous proliferation 135
Antiestrogens 98
Antifibrinolytic 51
Antiprogesterone 56
Antiprogestins 56
Anxiety 90
Aromatase inhibitors 56, 58, 63,
    103, 116, 120, 132
Artificial intelligence 137
Aseptic necrobiosis 46
Asherman syndrome 125
Asoprisnil 56, 58, 98, 116
Assisted reproductive
    technologies 12, 34
Atraumatic vascular bulldog
    clamps 74
Atrophy 45

B

Benign leiomyoma, typical 130
Beta-human chorionic
    gonadotropin 123
Bizarre nuclei 134
Bladder 112
Bleeding 82
  control of 68
  intermenstrual 42
  massive intraoperative 127
Blood
  loss 43
    reduce 74
  transfusion 73
  vessels 105
Bone mass 55
  index 6
Bone mineral density 52, 63, 115
Bonney clamp, application of 75*f*
Bonney myomectomy
    clamp 73, 74
Breast tenderness 51
Broad ligament 22, 72
  cysts 106
  fibroids 77

C

CA-125 105
Cabergoline 64
Caprini risk score 67
Cardiovascular problems 51
Cavity-distorting leiomyomas 34
Cell proliferation 10
Cellular
  atypia 137
  leiomyoma 134
Central cervical fibroid 110,
    111, 111*f*
Cervical cap placed 94
Cervical fibroid 22, 77, 89, 109
  anterolateral 112*f*
  enlarged 111*f*
  huge 110*f*
Cervical myoma 110
  diagnosis of 110
  enucleation of large 112
Cervix 72
Cesarean intramyometrial
    myomectomy 126
Cesarean myomectomy 127
  advantages of 127
  disadvantages of 127
  group 128
  indications for 126
Cesarean section 125, 128
  in pregnancy with fibroid 125
  tips and tricks for classical 126
  with fibroid 123, 126
Chemotherapy, role of 136
Cluster of differentiation 131
Coagulation disorders 42
Coagulative tumor necrosis 134
Coagulopathy 36*f*
Collagen type alpha 5, 9, 10
Combination oral
    contraceptives 64, 114
Combined hormonal
    contraception 48, 49,
    50, 51
Combined oral
    contraceptives 5, 114
Connective tissue 135
Contraceptives 14
Cornua 75
Counseling 77
Cryomyolysis 117, 118, 120
CYP19A1 encodes aromatase 10
Cystic degeneration 45

D

Dacarbazine 136
Danazol 59

Deaver retractors 73
Degeneration, features of 30
Demographic 4
   patterns 6
Diabetes 13, 14
Diarrhea 51
Diathermy, bipolar or monopolar 94
Dienogest 56
Diet 100
   and nutrition 13
   high-fat and high-calorie 13
Diffuse peritoneal leiomyomatosis 22
Digital health technologies 17
Dilatation and curettage 100
Dopamine agonist 62, 64
Dorsal lithotomy position 93
Doxorubicin 136
Drug, types of 50
Dysmenorrhea 98, 99
Dyspareunia 14, 91, 99
   feeling of pressure 110

E

Economic and healthcare factors 2
Elagolix 55, 56
Electrosurgical tip 76
Endocrine disruptors 13
Endocrine-disrupting chemicals 19
Endometrial
   ablation 53, 100
   biopsy 135
   bleeding 42
   cavity 75
      measuring 36f
   hyperplasia 114
   polyp 31f, 31
   stromal sarcoma 135
Endometrium 135
   distance and displacement of 29
Enzyme 10
Epidemiological methods, advancements in 16
Epithelioid tumors 136
Equine 55
Estradiol valerate 51
Estrogen 11, 55
   and progesterone, role of 11
   receptor 9
      alpha, production of 84

Ethnic and racial disparities 2, 7
Ethnicity and race 3
European Medicines Agency 57
Exercise 100
Exome sequencing 10
Extracellular matrix 20f
   regulation 10

F

Family planning and pregnancy 100
Fédération International de Gynécologie et d'Obstétrique 40, 41
Federation International Gynaecology and Obstetrics classification system 24
Female sexual function 89
Fertility 50
Fetal
   demise 124
   growth restriction 124
Fever 46, 77
Fibroblast growth factor, basic 41
Fibroid 24, 34, 35, 40, 48, 57, 73, 74f, 84, 93, 102, 123
   abnormal uterine bleeding with 40
   and subfertility 34
   cause of 1, 35
      pain during sex 89
   classification of 20
   diagnosis of 31
   effect on 85
      pregnancy on 123
   epidemiology and risk factors of 1
   impact fertility 34, 37
   in body of uterus 20
   in uterus 90f
   incidence of 5
   location of 41, 124
   management of 48, 53
      recurrent 96
   numbers of 19
   on pregnancy, effects of 124
   on quality of life, effect of 88
   polyp 42, 43
   presence of 88
   presurgical treatment of 62
   prevalence of 1, 2
   psychological impact of 89
   regrows 54

   related
      fertility 15
      pain 123
   removal, feasibility of 102
   risk factors for 8
   robotic-assisted management of 92
   secondary changes in 45
   size 50, 56
   small 62
   soft 24
   stiffness and rigidity of 24
   symptomatology of 40, 41t
   treatment of 88
   types of 35
   ultrasound mapping of 128
   uterus 19, 24f
      anatomical distributions of 21
      classification of 19
      Lasmar classification of 25f, 25t
      pathophysiology of 20f
   vessels 76f
   volume 73, 98
   with infertility, role of medical management of 38
Fluorodeoxyglucose 105
Follicle-stimulating hormone 85
   receptor 9
   secretion of 115
Food and Drug Administration 99, 115
Fruits and vegetables 13
Functional studies 10
Fundal fibroids 88
   intramural 21
   subserosal measuring 37f

G

Ganirelix 56
Gene, environment interactions 9
Genetic
   predisposition 3, 5
   susceptibility studies 10
Genetic syndromes 135
Genome-wide association studies 10
Genomic profiling 132
Gestrinone 59
Glycine, monopolar uses 81
Gonadotrophin-releasing hormone 37

Index

Gonadotropin hormone-releasing hormone 115, 120
  agonists 115
  antagonists inhibit 116
Gonadotropin receptors 53
Gonadotropin-releasing hormone 25, 42, 43, 49, 62, 81
  add-back therapy 63
  agonists 14, 50, 53, 54, 54*t*, 56, 62, 73, 103
    role of 73
  analogs 111, 132
  antagonist 14, 54, 55, 63
  receptor 56
  receptor blocker 56
Goserelin 53
Gravid uterus 128
Gynecological conditions, benign 102
Gynecologists, multidisciplinary team of 137

H

H-caldesmon 136
Health
  and quality of life, impact on 14
  disparities, impact on 8
  equity 2
Healthcare
  and diagnostic practices 3
  disparitie 4
  practices, changing 5
  utilization and economic burden 15
Healthy
  diet 15
  premenopausal women 56
Hemoglobin, preoperative 55
Hemorrhage 45, 77
  risk of 125
Hemostasis, complete 77
Herbal remedies 16
Hispanic 8
Histone deacetylase-8 136
Hormonal
  and lifestyle factors 3
  contraceptives 11
  factors 5, 11
  fluctuations and fibroid growth 11
  therapy 15, 96, 97*t*
    and fibroid risk 11

treatment 51
  preoperative 81
  presurgical 62
Hormone 104
  imbalances 90
  replacement therapy 11
  signaling 10
Hyaline degeneration 45
Hybrid 23
Hybrid fibroid 24
  ultrasound images of large 29*f*
Hydropic 45
Hyperplasia 36*f*
Hypertension 13
Hypoestrogenic 115
  state 63
Hypogastric plexus, inferior 89
Hypogonadotropic hypogonadal state 62
Hysterectomy 16, 55, 99, 115
  en bloc 136
  procedures 94
  unplanned 77
Hysterosalpingography 20
Hysteroscopic myomectomy 80, 82, 117
  complications of 82
  surgical technique of 80
Hysteroscopy 99
Hysterotomy incisions 126

I

Immunohistochemical markers 130
  stains like desmin 136
Immunohistochemistry 104
Immunotherapy in uterine sarcomas 137
In vitro fertilization 37
Incision, single/multiple 75
Indigestion 51
Infection 45, 77
Infertility 35
Infraumbilical midline vertical incision 126
Internal os 81
International Federation of Gynaecology and Obstetrics 26, 36*f*, 102
  abnormal uterine bleeding 29
  classification system 23, 117
    of fibroid uterus 23*f*
  staging for uterine sarcomas 136

subclassification for leiomyoma 41*f*
Interstitial 20
Intraligamentous location 69
Intramural 20, 43, 93
Intramural component 81
Intramural fibroid 35
  anterior 20
  large 28*f*
  posterior 21, 30*f*
Intramyometrial myomectomy 125
Intrauterine device 100
Intrauterine morcellator 82
Intrauterine system 49
  in fibroids 84
Intravenous leiomyomatosis 104
Intravenous oxytocin, use of 82

K

Ki-67 proliferation index 136

L

Lantern on top of St Paul's 110
Laparoendoscopic single-site surgery 70
Laparoscopic 117
  and open abdominal myomectomy 69
  cryomyolysis and thermocoagulation 117
  hysterectomy 99
  myomectomy 65, 69, 71, 103, 117
  procedures 65
  radiofrequency ablation 99
  surgery, advantages of 92
  suturing 66, 70
  techniques 93
    alternative 70
  thermocoagulation 118
  uterine artery occlusion 71
Laparotomy 69, 117
Lasmar classification of fibroid uterus 24
Layered closure 77
Leiomyomas 28, 34, 36*f*, 38, 40, 46, 65, 72, 96, 102, 103, 114, 123, 134
  atypical 134
  classification of 29
  in sonography 28
  subserosal 66*f*

symptomatic intramural 66f
types of 134
Leiomyomatosis peritonealis
disseminata 104
Leiomyosarcoma 32, 135
diagnosis 135
etiology 135
histopathology 135
malignant 130
management 136
prognosis 137
Lesions, benign 45
Letrozole 56, 58, 116
Leuprolide acetate 53
Levonorgestrel intrauterine
system 43, 48, 50, 52, 64
Levonorgestrel-releasing
intrauterine system 53,
115, 120
Lifestyle and environmental
factors 12
Lifestyle factors 4
Lifestyle modifications 100
Li–Fraumeni syndrome 135
Linea alba 74f
Lipoleiomyomas 32
Liver metastasis 106
Luteinizing hormone 85, 115
secretion 62
Lymph node 105, 136
positivity 137
Lymphadenectomy 136
Lymphovascular channels 137

M

Magnetic resonance imaging 20,
80, 110, 131
guided focused
ultrasound 48, 118
surgery 16, 38, 49, 120
high-frequency 118
Malignancy 36f, 137
Marked nuclear atypia 135
Matrix metalloproteinase, level
of 41
Mediator complex subunit 9
Medicated intrauterine system 52
Medicine Agency of European
Union 99
Medicines and Healthcare
products Regulatory
Agency 58
Medroxyprogesterone
acetate 52, 115

Mefenamic acid 51
Menarche 12
Menopausal symptoms 63
Menstrual
bleeding 8
heavy 40, 41, 48, 56,
65, 88, 130
blood loss 98
flow 115
irregularities 14
Metabolic syndrome 14
Metastasis systems 136
Metastasizing leiomyoma,
benign 105
Mifepristone 56, 58, 63, 97, 116
Minimally invasive gynecological
surgeries 92, 99
Mirena 52
Mitotic rate 137
Mitotically active leiomyoma 134
Monoclonal tumors 48
Monopolar electrosurgical
instrument 76
Morcellation 68, 94, 132
Morcellators 117
Morphological uterus
sonographic 26
Multi-omic data, integration of 17
Musa consensus 25, 26t
Muscular tissue 105
Myocardin point 136
Myolysis 65
Myoma 65, 68f, 72, 102, 114,
116, 123
ablation of 82
challenging 81
dissection 67
evaluation of 80
removal of 76, 116
separation 68f
shelling of 76
volume, reduction in 119
Myomectomy 16, 70, 93, 99,
115, 117, 120
clamp 76
use of 74f
in pregnancy, role of 124
on pregnancy 125
screw 73
Myometrial
echogenicity 26
incision 26, 67
myoma junction, necrosis
of 73

Myometrium 48, 93
overlying 67
wall of 26
Myxoid 45

N

National Institute for Health
and Care Excellence
guideline 57
Nausea 46
Necrobiosis, prevent 126
Necrosis 45
Neodymium-doped yttrium–
aluminum–garnet 82
Nondecent vaginal
hysterectomy 49
Nonhormonal treatment 50
Nonsteroidal anti-inflammatory
drugs 14, 48, 49, 50,
82, 98
Nonsteroidal estrogen receptor
ligands 116
Norethisterone acetate 52

O

OBE-2109 59
Obesity 6, 13
and physical activity 13
Oligomenorrhea 53
Onapristone 116
Oophorectomy 137
Open abdominal
myomectomy 72
Open myomectomy 78
use instruments for 73
Oral contraceptive pills 64, 120
Oral progestogens 52
Ormeloxifene 56, 58
Ovarian
reserve 118
tumors 106
Ovulatory dysfunction 36f

P

p53 136
Pain
and pressure during sex 90
in abdomen 118
management 77
severe 46
Para-aortic lymph node
dissection 136

Parasitic 102
    fibroids 22, 102, 105, 107, 117
    leiomyoma 104
        management of 106
        variants of 103
    myomas 103
Parity 12
    and pregnancy 12
Pazopanib 136
Pedunculated 21
    fibroids 22, 85, 93
    submucous fibroids 35
    subserosal myomas 103
    subserous fibroid 22, 107
Pelvic
    pain 65, 91, 98
        and pressure 14
    pressure 98
    region of women 84
    structures, lateral 111f
    tumors 106
Perimenopausal
    age-group 91
    menorrhagia 114
    transition 7
Peritoneal structure 46
Pesticides and herbicides 13
Pfannenstiel incision 49, 74f
Placenta 124
    implantation of 125
Polygenic inheritance 9
Polypoidal myomas 109
Port placement 67
Positron emission
        tomography 104
Postmenopausal period 7
Postpartum complications 124
Potential metastasis 104
Pouch of Douglas 110
Predominant neoplasms 84
Preeclampsia 124
Pregnancy 12
    hormones, changes in 123
    specific parameters 30
    with fibroid 125
Preterm
    birth 128
    prelabor rupture of
        membranes 124
Proellex 98
Progesterone 11, 132
    absence of 84
    receptors 62, 116
        expression of 84
        modulator 57

Progestins 62, 63, 114, 120
Progestogens 52
    high-dose oral 52
    injectable 52
Prophylactic antibiotics 67
    role of 73
    use of 67
Pseudocapsule 34
    with monopolar tip 76f
Pseudofibroid 22
Pseudo-Meig syndrome 22
Pseudomenopause 62, 115
Psychosexual dysfunction, cause
        of 89
Psychosocial problems 88

Q

Quality of life 48, 72
    impact on 15

R

Racial and ethnic disparities 5
Radiofrequency
    ablation 38, 49
    fibroid ablation 70, 71
Raloxifene 55
Red degeneration 46
    pathology of 46
    symptoms of 46
    treatment of 46
Red meat and dairy 13
Regular exercise 15
Relugolix 56
Relugolix-Estradiol-
        norethisterone
        acetate 59
Renal cell carcinoma 106
Reproductive factors 3, 12
Reproductive issues 14
Research
    advancing 2
    challenges and
        opportunities 16
Retroperitoneal lymph node
        dissection, role of 136
Retroperitoneum 105
Reversible contraceptive,
        long-acting 50
Robotic-assisted laparoscopy 93
Robotic surgery 92
    advantages and drawbacks
        of 93
Rupture of myomectomy scar 77

S

Saline infusion sonography 20,
        28, 31, 80
Saponification 46
Sarcoma, undifferentiated 135
Sarcomatous changes 45
Scalpel 76
Sedation 46
Selective estrogen receptor
        modulator 11, 55, 56,
        62, 63, 103, 116, 120
Selective progesterone receptor
        modulator 48, 56, 62,
        63, 97, 116, 120
Serosa, closed baseball suture 76f
Serosal contour 26
Sessile fibroids 22
Sexual and psychosexual
        dysfunction 88
Shear wave elastography score 24
Single-port laparoscopy 70, 71
Skin incision 73
Slicing technique 81
Smooth muscle
    actin 136
    cells 48, 93, 105
    origin 136
    tumor
        benign 109
        of uncertain malignant
            potential 105, 134, 135
        spectrum 131
Socioeconomic and healthcare
        access factors 8
Space-occupying lesions 91
Spotting 53
STEP-W classification 81t
    and management of
        fibroids 42t
    of fibroid uterus 24, 25t
    of submucous fibroid 25t
Stress management 15, 100
Submucosal 41, 93
    fibroids 22, 24t, 25, 31, 42f,
        85, 89
    myoma 109
Subserosal 93, 103
    anterior wall fibroid
        measuring 37f
    fibroid 46, 103, 124, 125
        anterior 21
        posterior 22

Suctioning 94
Systemic inflammatory response syndrome 77

T

Tamoxifen 63
Telapristone 98, 116
Temozolomide 136
Temporary atraumatic vascular clamp 74
Tenaculum 68*f*
Thermocoagulation 117, 120
Thromboprophylaxis 67, 77
Tibolone 55
Tissue retraction 94
Tissue-specific effects 116
Touching endometrium 29
Tourniquet 73
Trabectedin 136
Tranexamic acid 16, 51, 98
　functions 51
　indications of 51
Transforming growth factor-beta, synthesis of 96
Transient myometrial contractions 32
Transvaginal ultrasound 30, 20, 80, 106
Triptorelin 53
Tumors
　benign 45, 80, 102, 103, 114, 135
　prevalent 96
　infiltrates abdominal tissues 136
　malignant 135
　types of 135

U

Ulipristal 63, 116
Ulipristal acetate 37, 56, 98
Ultrasonography, three-dimensional 30
Ureter 112
Ureteral stenting, bilateral 112
Urinary
　symptoms 14
　tract infection 41
Uterine
　artery 65
　　embolization 16, 38, 48, 49, 99, 111, 117, 118, 120
　　occlusion 118, 120
　　resistance index 85
　bleeding
　　abnormal 40, 50, 99, 110, 115, 134
　　with fibroids, abnormal 41
　cavity entry 68, 69*f*
　cervix 109
　defects, closure of 66, 68
　fibroids 2, 9, 20*f*, 28, 65, 72, 85, 88, 96, 102, 104, 109, 114, 115
　　classification 21
　　diagnosis of 28
　　incidence patterns of 4
　　management of 49*f*
　　multifaceted nature of 65
　　pathophysiology of 20
　　symptomatic 88, 114
　leiomyomas, treatment of 65
　myomas 80, 106
　natural killer cells 34
　preserving
　　surgical modalities 117
　　treatment modalities 114
　rupture, increased risk of 69
　sarcomas 135
　smooth muscle tumors 130
　　of uncertain malignant potential 130
　　spectrum of 130
　soft-tissue tumors 131
　vessels 75*f*, 75, 112
Uterus 24, 26, 30*f*, 72
　and ovarian tourniquet 74
　exteriorizing 73
　image of 32*f*
　incision over 75
　innervation of 89*f*
　preserving treatment modalities 119*f*, 120
　sitting 109*f*
　surgical removal of 93

V

Vaginal
　bleeding 46
　hysterectomy 99
　occlusion of uterine arteries 119
Vaporization 82
Vascular
　changes 45
　clamps 73
Vasopressin 67, 74
　use of 75
Venous thromboembolism 55
Vessel clips 112
Vomiting 46

W

Wamsteker classification 24*t*, 25
　of submucous fibroid 24
Wandering fibroid 22, 102
　epidemiology 102
　managing 103
　pathogenesis and etiology 103
Weight gain 52
White women, lower prevalence in 8
Whole-genome sequencing 10
Wilms tumor 131
WNT ligands 96